Canimalism

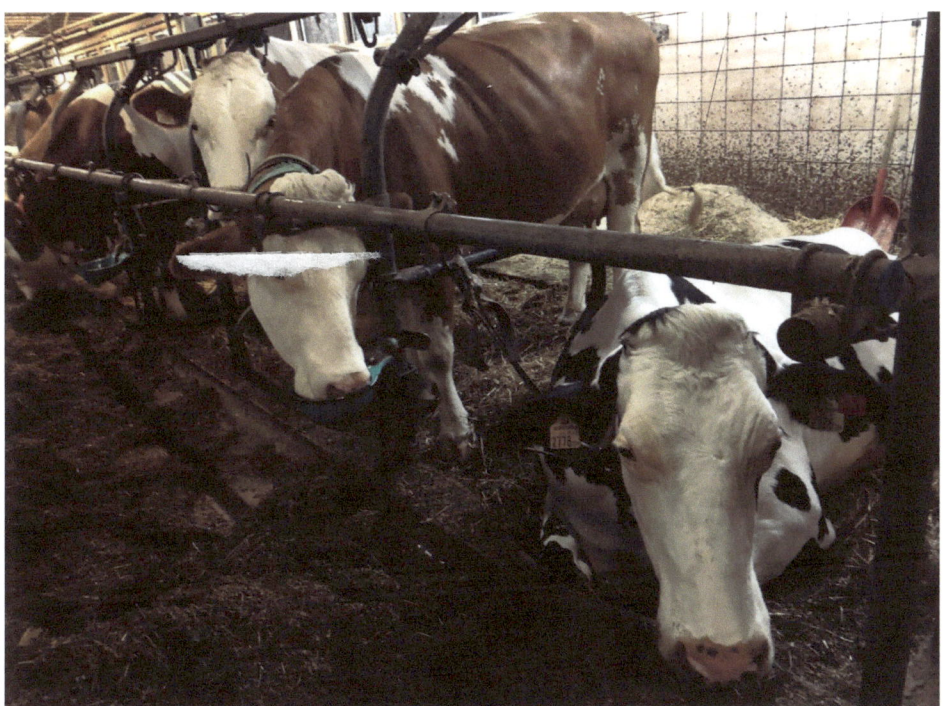

September 21, 2019.

Copyright © 2019 Dr. Peter A.J. Holst

120 pages

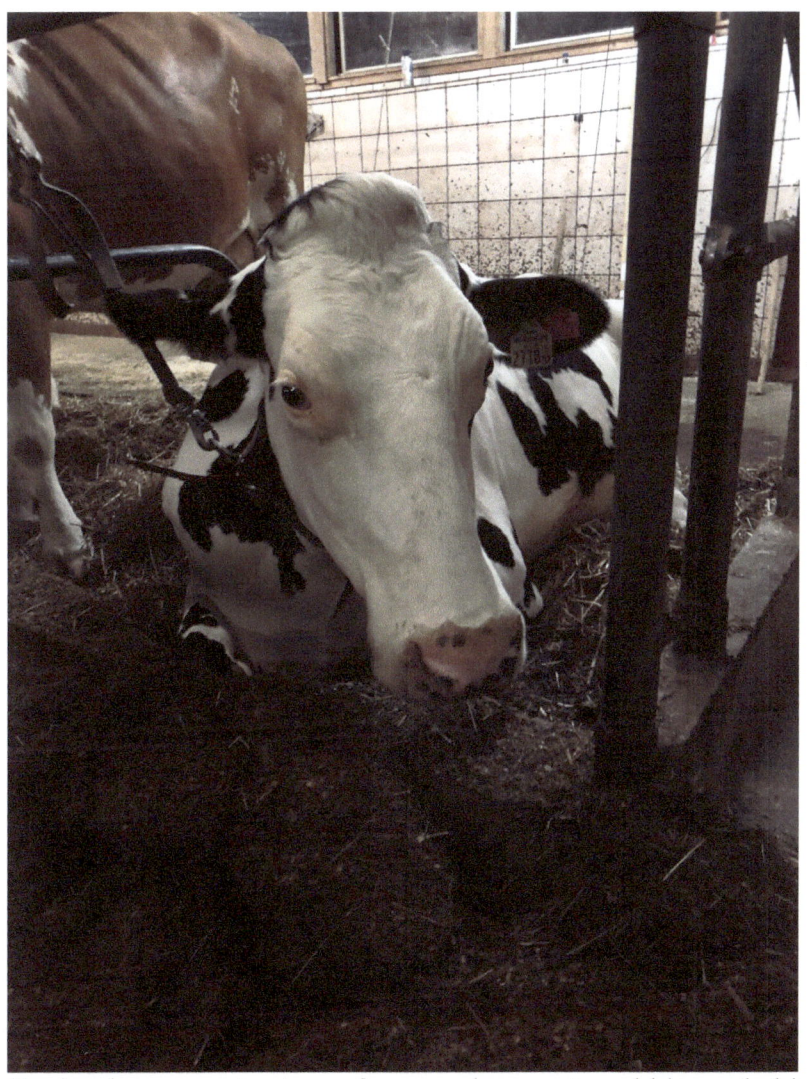

Canimals are meat eaters of cows, pigs, goats, rabbits and chickens that have been intensively bred for consumption.

Biography

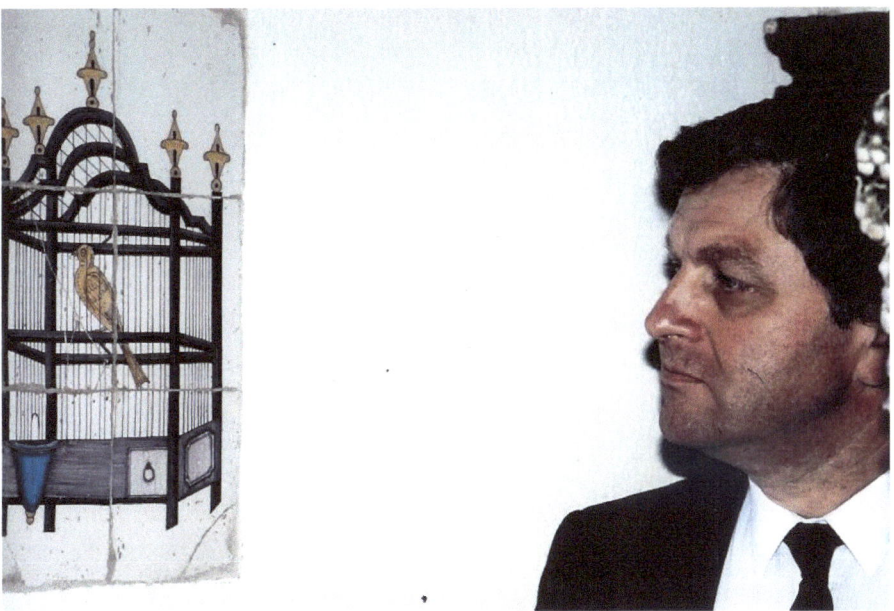

Peter A.J. Holst went to study health care at the University of Utrecht. At this university, lectures and practice were combined at the faculties of human medicine, veterinary medicine and dentistry until the candidate exam. At the student association he was soon informed that he did not study health care but medicine. A first excursion to Paris was financed by the pharmaceutical industry. At the l'Oree du Bois de Boulogne we were received princely in a Michelin restaurant. From now on, no patient should leave the consulting room without a prescription.
For the bachelor examination of the bachelor he did his pathology exam with Professor A. de Minjer. His thesis on small cell lung cancer

was discussed and the Minjer took him to the pottery museum where they stopped for some time in front of a preparation with lung carcinoma of a smoker. De Minjer pointed out to him that lung cancer and breast cancer for the coming years would be the biggest challenges of medicine. More than fifty years later, that is still the case.

After assistantships in Rotterdam and Leiden, he graduated from the University of Leiden in 1969. During the midwifery internship in Leiden, Professor A. Sikkel asked him to assist in the practice of Dr. P.J. Meijst in Hazerswoude. In the event of a collision on the provincial road, this general practitioner had broken his shoulder and had to be assisted for several months in the practice. An additional advantage was that during this period there would certainly be some deliveries where I could assist. That came true because during my assistantship I could lead more home deliveries than I could have done in the obstetric clinic in Leiden. Professor Sikkel has made contraception an indispensable part of the profession and, has institutionalized the establishment of a separate outpatient clinic for contraception. Professor Sikkel was a very inspiring doctor.

Holst worked as a general practitioner in Rijswijk-Den Haag from 1970 to 1984. In his early years as a general practitioner, Holst was also supervisor of a clinic for birth control in Delft (Dr. Rutgers Foundation) for several years. The Rutgers Foundation was successful in the seventies of the twentieth century with its counseling agencies for contraception, the Rutgershuizen. In 1969 and 1970 he held evening office hours at the Rutgershuis in Delft. When the St Hippolytus hospital on the Phoenixstraat in Delft moved to a new location, the former hospital was transformed into a business collection building. Under the direction of Holst, the incubator department on the top floor of this building was converted into a number of consultation and examination rooms of the new Rutgershuis in Delft. He has placed about 250 IUDs in all of the following practical years, including in his own general practice during evening consultation hours for contraception and cervical smears. He held back-guard consultation hours for the morning after pill. Real 'Hagueneses' then asked for the "morning after save pill".

Under influence of the Nederlands Huisartsen Instituut, his practice was set up from the beginning with a surveillance schedule. This means that age groups are always tested for the risks that occur in the age group. As additional operations during consultation contacts at least once the blood pressure was measured, for example also once from 50 years the eye pressure measured and noted, the stool examined for occult blood loss from 50 years, in risk groups also an electrocardiogram was made, etc. At the beginning of my general practice, I found a severe pneumonia in a young woman of 20 years old. After treatment with an antibiotic she recovered. Because she had a cage with a parakeet in her bedroom, I wondered whether the presence of a cage bird in the house could possibly cause more serious illness. A 17 years old boy died of bone cancer in his leg during the first years of my practice. This young man had constantly kept and bred at least 100 tropical songbirds in a basement. One can imagine the risk of repeated bird flu and the occurrence of blood and bone marrow episodes with slow-moving carcinogenic bone infection in such intensive contact. Because of the many consultation hours and home visits, ten lung cancer patients came to my attention in a year. Of these, there were six bird keepers in the years before diagnosis. After consulting with professor F. de Waard of the RIVM, department of epidemiology, I have set up a ten-year practice survey and follow-up studies. The statistical link was demonstrated, later confirmed in studies in Berlin and Glasgow. Much later, in 2012 a laboratory experiment proved the link between lung cancer and Chlamydia pneumonia infection.

In 1987, this research led to his PhD at the University of Utrecht on the relationship he demonstrated between breeding and keeping birds indoors and lung cancer. He defended the hypothesis that lung cancer in bird keepers and bird breeders is the result of persistent infection of the deeper basal cells in the airways. His promoters were prof. F. de Waard, epidemiologist of the RIVM, professor P. Zwart, special veterinary faculty and D. Kromhout, nutritional epidemiologist.

These basal cells, also called cancer stem cells, are still multipotent and do not die if the cell is infected with a bacterium like the Chlamydia that can only propagate in a living host cell. The practical studies and the dust measurements with TNO were supported by the Dutch Prevention Fund. After this he started working as director of Health, Safety and Environment services.

After his retirement in 2005, he started traveling a lot. Born in Zeeland (1943), on land in the sea, the sea-hole and the wide world continued to attract him. He has crossed all the oceans several times.

Foreword to the Original Studies

Original ideas and observations are rare. They are especially valuable if checked in practice, critically evaluated and supported by material independently collected by others.
It is to the very personal credit of Dr. P.A.J. Holst that he noticed a potential connection between the keeping of birds and the occurrence of lung cancer among members of households where they are kept. He has pursued the idea in his private practice and for over 12 years kept records of every single patient. The data were critically and statistically analysed and supplemented by data and materials collected by lung specialists.
A new aspect is presented in this book. Avian products, spread in the house in the form of fine dust particles, may be inhaled deeply, cause irritation and contribute to local immune response in the lungs. It is hypothesized that this sequence of events is independent of other factors and significantly contributes to lung cancer and some other diseases.
It is a pleasure to work with a gifted man who is fascinated by many aspects of human well being. The author is well aware of the importance of contact between mankind and nature. Living creatures such as dogs, cats, pet and aviary birds play a major role in human well being. The keeping of birds may, however, as many other activities, also brings certain health risks. Holst analyses the habits of bird keepers and the consequences of bird keeping on the health of residents of houses where birds are kept. This book is a condensed presentation of an important scientific work contributing significantly to the health and well-being of mankind.

Professor P. Zwart DVM PhD
University of Utrecht, the Netherlands

Follow-up Intensive Breeding of Animals

Darwin wondered after comparative studies on the Galapagos Islands - The Origin of Species - what his findings meant for the further evolution of life on Earth.

- Charles Darwin showed that the finches on isolated Galapagos islands developed under the influence of their environment.

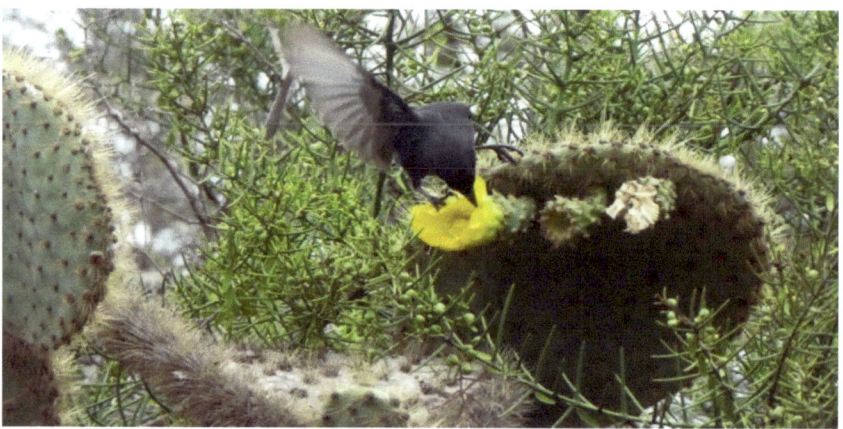

- **Darwin showed that environmental factors translate into physical and genetic characteristics.**

From their tree huts in Africa, the great apes developed a great hand skill. About a million years ago chimpanzees reached the warmer areas of Europe and Asia. From Africa through the Middle East, 60,000 years ago hominids reached Asia (*Homo luzonensis* and *floresiensis*) and 45.000 years ago Western Europe (*Homo neanderthalis*).
People, chimpanzees and gorillas shared a common ancestor up to 5 million years ago.

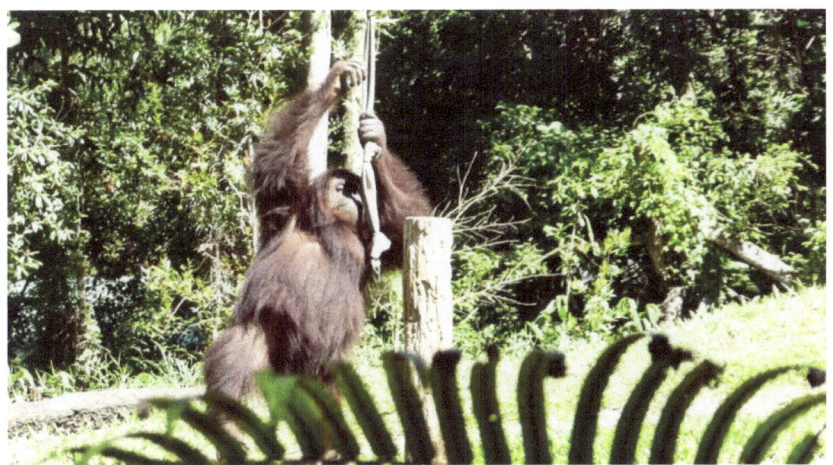

(Alfred Russel Wallace. The Malay Archipelago, land of the Orangutan and the bird of paradise)

The orangutan has no tail and walk on two legs. Great apes have started to walk upright, on two legs. Standing, it is easier to gaze at prey or enemies, and arms that are not needed for locomotion remain free for other purposes, such as throwing stones or giving signals. Homo sapiens has achieved greater dexterity in the East African region. Man is the only man-like person who can place the thumb against the other fingers and make a precision grip with his hands. The more those hands were able to do, the more successful their owners were, so the evolutionary pressure led to an increasing concentration of nerves and extremely precise muscles in the thumb and fingers. The brain grew with it. As a result, people can perform particularly complex tasks with their hands. Only modern man, due to the increased volume of the brain, has been able to control the reproductive processes and to free himself from the instinctive process of reproduction in the mid-twentieth century. Consumption animals are badly off with this new knowledge.

Artificial insemination techniques are also the result of this new insight. The increase in meat products and dairy production in the West could only be achieved with manual insemination of mammals and the animals unilaterally fattening with soy flour, corn and fish meal.

The unbridled breeding of animals, through artificial insemination of cattle and with incubators for poultry, has a devastating effect on our health, nature and the climate. Fast food, unnatural food and meat consumption lead to obesity, vitamin deficiencies, chronic diseases and premature death. Cancer is now the main cause of premature death.

- Since the second half of the 20th century, modern humans have eradicated 60% of mammals, birds, fish and reptiles in the wild.
- Agricultural subsidies break down the grasslands.
- Fuel subsidies for the major fish trawlers destroy the fish stocks of the oceans.
- We can no longer ignore the impact of current non-sustainable production models.

Index
Page
- 14. Introduction
- 18. Diseases in humans due to intensive farming
- 27. Employee risks in the meat industry
- 29. Employee risks in the poultry industry
- 33. Diseases later in life resulting from fast food
- 46. Dairy industry
- 47. Raw egg proteins and raw milk products
- 49. Why people have become carnivores
- 51. Fishmeal industry

- 53. Bowel cancer
- 56. Breast cancer
- 63. Lung cancer
- 67. Experimental induction of lung cancer
- 74. Trade in tropical birds and pigeons
- 80. Tobacco industry

- 83. Global warming
- 85. Desertification on 2/3 of all the land on earth
- 87. Wildlife loss
- 89. Overpopulation

- 91. Hydrogen as energy source offers the solution
- 99. Farming transition offers the solution
- 103. Let plant-based food be the medicine for health
- 110. Simply make your own meals
- 114. References

Introduction

The interest in the connection shown by the author between breeding tropical birds and lung cancer has expanded to the health risks of the intensive breeding of poultry, pigs and cattle for consumption. Since the fifties of the 20th century, intensive breeding in livestock has increased sharply. An increase that keeps pace with the recent increase in cancer mortality.

In the past many large and small mammals have been domesticated. The population has acquired immunity against the great epidemics of the past. Zoonotic infections like the black plague, smallpox, tuberculosis, measles, typhoid and cholera could be treated with vaccination and antibiotics.

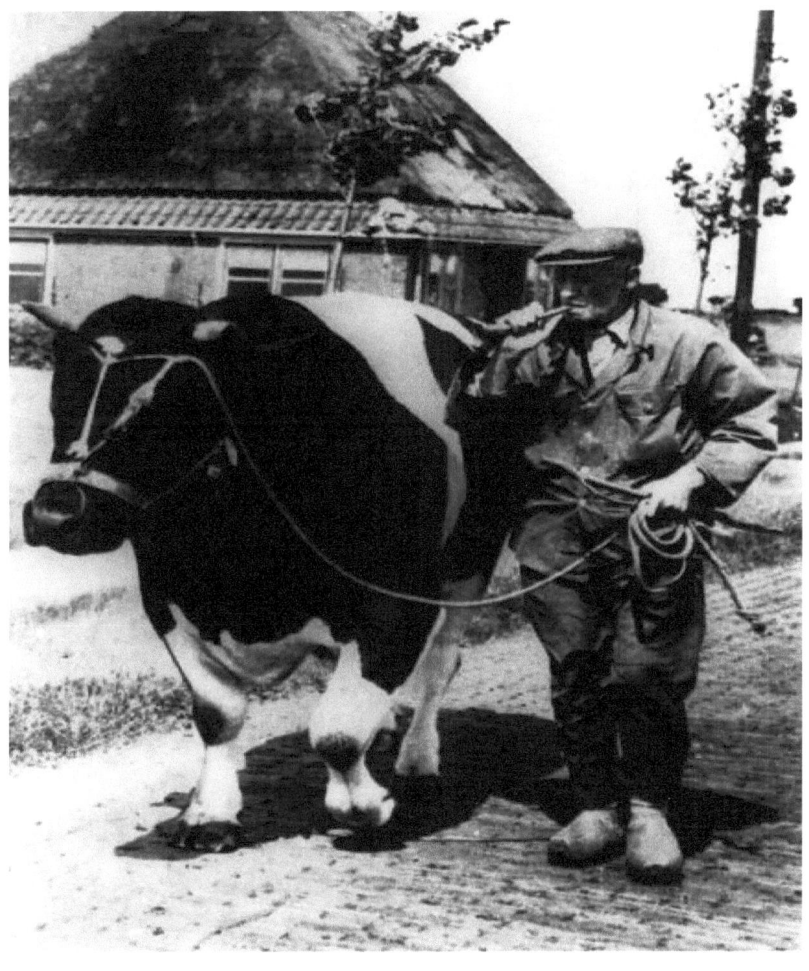

Less than a hundred years ago the bull runner with the bull went to the farms where a cow had to be covered.

Since the middle of the twentieth century we have a new situation, caused by intensive farming. All meat of farmed mammals is only produced by manual insemination of cattle, pigs and rabbits. Mad cow disease, swine fever and bird flu are the result of intensive livestock farming.

Harmful consequences of artificial insemination of livestock for health and climate

The population explosion and famine on earth have caused man to artificially inseminate animals and to breed exclusively for consumption. Fast food and an increase in meat consumption in the West are simulated in other parts of the world. Fast food, unnatural food and hamburger consumption lead to obesity and chronic diseases. In the meantime, the number of cancer diseases is increasing and is nowadays prime cause of chronic diseases and premature death in the elderly. The ceiling for meat and meat products has already been reached with the current 7 billion world population. The production of meat (products), poultry, pork and other meat tripled between 1980 and 2010 and is expected to double again in 2050

- 50 years of artificial insemination in mammals

The increase in meat and dairy products is only achieved with artificial insemination of cattle. The production of milk, cheese and meat is inextricably linked. The cow must give birth to as many calves as possible for milk, cheese and meat. Female calves grow up to be dairy cows, bulls go to the meat industry. As a result, carcinogenic viruses are now found in cattle and in the meat and dairy industry. Harmful viruses such as Avian (poultry) leukemia virus (ALV) and Bovine (cattle) leukemia virus (BLV) are found in raw egg proteins and meat products. Harmful leukemia viruses from cattle and poultry have spread to animal caretakers, employees in the meat and poultry industry and consumers (Johnson 2010, Blair 1982).

Global warming is largely the result of intensive livestock production. During the last ice age man was forced to eat more meat because there were fewer grains, fruits, nuts and seeds. Will modern man eat more vegetable food now that the earth is warming up?
The pig used to be kept as a food reserve for the cold winter months. Hams and sausages etc. We have started to eat more meat without fruit and vegetables. The theme of "artificial reproduction in mammals for increasing meat production" has never been brought before. Making livestock farming more sustainable is certainly not going to work to prevent global warming and the loss of plant and animal species. To make this book not only a message of doom I do proposals for more plant food and farming transition.

The farmers can repurpose their stalls with a power plant for heat and LED lighting. Strawberries, mushrooms, peppers, lettuce, grapes and pineapples can now also be produced in winter. With local production with a greater supply and diversity, the supply of fruit and vegetables over the equator will decrease.

Diseases in humans due to intensive farming

Our dealings with mammals have been going on for thousands of years since we domesticated them. Infectious diseases that occur in animals mainly spread when large numbers of animals are brought together. A disease can then spread over the entire herd. Many farmers live close to their cattle and come into contact with their droppings, urine, breath, ulcers and blood. A disease can thus turn to humans and reach epidemic proportions if a group of people first come into contact with such a disease.

In the early Middle Ages (14th century) grain stocks of farmers in Mongolia attracted rats, marmots and mice. Rats and their fleas passed Pasteurella pestis (bubonic plague and lung plague) to the local population. The steppe marmot is the most common reservoir for Pasteurella pestis in East Asia. The meat was eaten from the marmots and the skins were processed into fur. During the siege by the Mongols of the Genoese trading office Kaffa, on the Black Sea, hundreds of bodies of victims of the plague with catapults were shot in the besieged city to infect residents with plague. Genoese sailors were struck by the plague in 1345. Survivors and sick fled with their ships from the city to Sicily and Genoa. The Genoese fleet first contaminated the inhabitants of Messina in Sicily. From Genoa, the disease spread through the extensive trade network of Europe. The disease was spread throughout Europe.

- **The bubonic plague and lung plague killed 25 million people, 50% of the European population, in the 14th century.**

Cristobal Colon (Columbus) was born in Genoa, and more sailors from Genoa were undoubtedly signed on the ships of the explorers.

They knew the history of this manner of warfare. In the conquest of South America, the Spaniards brought new diseases with them. Ironically, the only epidemic that Europeans brought back from South America was the syphilis, a not so enjoyable sexually transmitted disease.

- **Smallpox and tuberculosis have wiped out entire civilizations in South America in the 16th century.**

An Influenza A(viary) virus caused a flu epidemic in Fort Riley, Kansas. In this fort they bred chickens and pigs for the soldiers. A cook might have been infected with the virus. By mutation, the virus was able to bring about contagion from person to person.

- **The new bird flu virus (H1N1) was transferred by the troop transports in WW1 from the USA to Europe with millions of deaths as a result.**

Factory farming

The discovery of antibiotics and vaccines made it possible to keep cattle in large numbers. According to the BBC, the era of intensive livestock farming in Great Britain began in 1947. An agricultural law subsidized the farmers to stimulate production with new technology and to reduce Britain's dependence on meat imports. At the end of the last century, sheep heads containing prion particles from diseased animals were given to British cows. Natural herbivores - cows that eat grass and hay - were turned into carnivores, which ate meat and bone flour instead of grass, for faster growth and more financial gain. This caused the mad cow disease (BSE) due to damage to the brain and bones in the cow. The disease later also caused a variant of this in humans.

- **Mad cow disease (BSE) is spread by contaminated meat.**

Laying hens

A study of 466 laying hens, ranging from 2 to 7 years, over a period of more than 3 years, has yielded data on reproductive organs and tumor formation in laying hens. Laying hens get ovarian cancer, but these tumors are rare in hens for the second year of life. At the commercial poultry farms, chickens are usually sacrificed after laying their first year, no later than 22-24 months old. Occasionally these hens reach a second leg year. Most cancers occur in these hens. The belly of the hens swells up due to fluid accumulation and the tumors are tangibly present. Of the 466 hens in this study, 149 (32%) developed ovarian tumors. The number of ovarian tumors was 39 (8%). In addition, 22 hens (5%) received benign swellings from the supporting tissue of the fallopian tube. In total, 45% of these laying hens received tumors from the reproductive organs.

- **Ovarian and ovarian cancer is most common in hens above the age at which most are slaughtered**

Chicken meat is highly contaminated

Every year, 45 billion chickens pass the world, along with 1 billion pigs, who can have contact with an estimated 50 billion waterfowl, such as ducks, geese and swans. Never before has the highly contagious avian flu, the influenza A avian flu virus, had such a chance to spread. Broiler chickens are bred to grow quickly in weight (Deshazo RD). In 1920 a chicken reached 1 kg in 16 weeks. The current broiler chickens now reach a weight of 2.6 kg, large enough for slaughter, in just 6 weeks. Over the past 50 years, growth has increased from 25 grams to 100 grams per day - an increase of more than 300%. Genetic selection is so intense that the age at which broilers reach their market weight and are slaughtered has dropped by as much as one day per year. Selection for rapid growth has resulted in poor health of the bones, causing deformities, lameness, tibia dyschondroplasia (TD) and ruptured tendons. Heavier broilers (> 2400 g) are often crippled. Sometimes the birds are no longer able to walk at all. Broilers and chicken products are heavily contaminated with antibiotic-insensitive (multi-resistant) Escherichia Coli and are considered as a source of human infections. The percentage of infected chickens in Dutch broiler farms increased in the first week of life from 0-24% to 96-100%, regardless of the use of antibiotics and remained 100% up to slaughter (Dierikx CM). Multidrug-resistant intestinal bacteria were found in turkeys, cattle, chickens and retail meat products in Oklahoma. Sample were insensitive to commonly used antibiotics such as ampicillin, tetracycline, streptomycin, gentamycin and kanamycin. In Germany, multi resistant staphylococci (MRSA) were detected in samples of turkey (40%) and broilers (25%), also in pig farms, with higher frequencies in fattening farms (73%) than in breeding farms (33%). Pork and chicken meat are potentially sources of multi resistant species.

- **More antibiotics are provided to livestock than to humans**.

The increasing availability of antibiotics in the 1950s and 1960s was the reason to predict the 'beginning of the end' for infections. Nothing is further from the truth! Insensitivity to antibiotics increases and the arrival of new antibiotics decreases. Whatever the pharmaceutical industry is trying to do, there is no doubt that the microorganisms that have already existed for 3 billion years have adapted to survive under the most extreme conditions. Bloody diarrhea after eating insufficiently heated chicken or pork, for example after a barbecue, is a dangerous phenomenon. In some cases, bloody diarrhea is caused by multidrug-resistant Coli bacteria. Especially in women, these gut bacteria reach the bladder. The bacteria attach to the bladder wall and hardly respond to treatment with antibiotics. The urine becomes bloody. Not infrequently, these bacteria go higher and reach the kidneys through the ureter.

- **Entero hemolytic E. coli bacteria (EHEC) can cause severe kidney failure**.

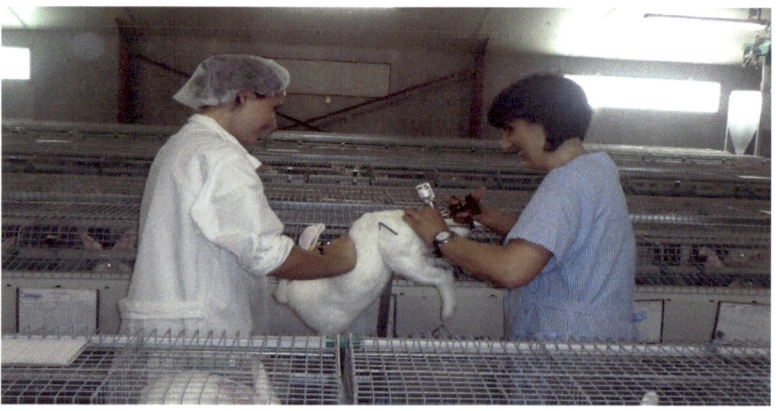

Rabbits are the second most bred animals in Europe

Female rabbits kept for breeding have specific problems. Those that are not used to feed the young are given little food and are often starved. On average, female rabbits are artificially inseminated 11 days after delivery. The impact of such a burden on their bodies is devastating, resulting in illness and death. More than 330 million rabbits are bred each year (more than all pigs and EU cows together). Every year more than a billion rabbits are slaughtered worldwide - most for their meat, a few for their fur. China accounts for about half that number, but the EU slaughters more than 326 million rabbits annually, especially in France, Spain and Italy. Most of them live in a small space. The majority is crammed in bare sheds with between 10,000 and 20,000 animals. The amount of space that is usually allowed for each rabbit is less than an A4 sheet of paper. While a well-groomed rabbit will live for about eight years or longer, rabbits reared for the meat are slaughtered at just three months of age. Of course they can hop about 70 cm, but most commercially grown rabbits are not able to jump or sit up straight, instead of being able to jump. Because of the low height of their cages, some cannot even light their ears.

- **Hepatitis E virus (HEV) strains of reared rabbits indicate that these mammals can be a reservoir for HEVs that cause infection in humans.**

BBQ meat and hepatitis E virus

One in ten sausages and processed pork products in England and Wales can cause a hepatitis E virus (HEV) infection if the meat is not done, experts warn. Sausages must be cooked for 20 minutes at 70 degrees Celsius to kill the virus. There has been an "abrupt increase" in the number of cases in England and Wales, because people do not realize the risk. Hepatitis E is a liver infection that is spread by direct contact with fecal material from an infected person or by indirect fecal contamination of food or water sources. Pregnant women who become infected are at greater risk of acute liver failure, loss of the child and death.

Artificial Insemination

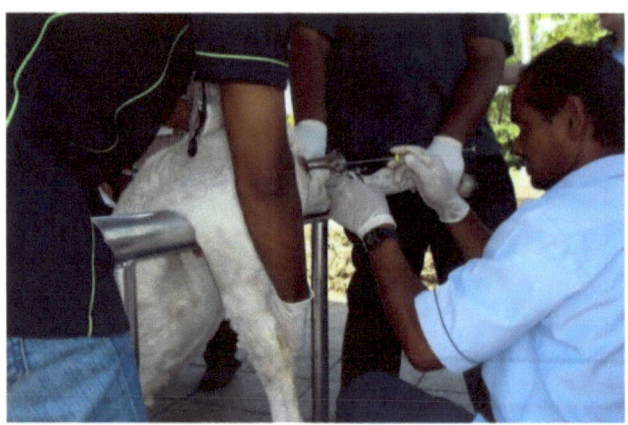

Intensive goat domestication and Q fever
Manure and straw from the goats are distributed by farmers as fertilization over the land. As a result, the Coxiella bacterium spreads through the air and infects the local population (Schimmer B).

Severe Acute Respiratory Syndrome (SARS)
SARS was caused by a corona virus and originated in South China province Guangdong (Canton) in November 2002. The worldwide outbreak of SARS was triggered on one day in a hotel in Hong Kong from a single person. A doctor from Guangdong participated in a grand wedding party. When the guests left, the virus, coughed up by this doctor, spread to five countries within 24 hours. In a few months, this coronavirus spread to 30 countries on six continents, producing 8,096 probable cases and 774 deaths (WHO 2004). In the past a trip

around the world took a year; today, we with our viral luggage can travel around the earth in 24 hours. The Guangdong authorities cleared thousands of civet cats and other wild animals in January 2004. They also imposed a permanent ban on the trade and human consumption of civet cats. Researchers showed that humans and civet cats had viruses with the same genetic profile, after testing six SARS-carrying civet cats from a restaurant. At the beginning of 2004, a waitress was infected by the SARS virus. WHO experts also demonstrated the virus in cages of a restaurant where a SARS patient had eaten meat from civet cats. Unfortunately, Chinese people prefer a large range of wild animals, and the civet cat is considered a delicacy in South China. In rural China, the animals are still sold on the markets.

Dromedary flu (MERS-CoV)
Dromedary flu, from virus-spreading young camels, is the result of intensive camel breeding on the Arabian Peninsula. There is a rapid increase in the number of reported infections with Middle East Respiratory Syndrome Corona Virus (MERS-CoV). Since June 2012, MERS-CoV has infected more than 1,814 people, including 734 deaths (41%). The disease first appeared on the Arabian Peninsula, in Saudi Arabia and the United Arab Emirates. Concerns about the situation have increased considerable, particularly concerns about the spread of the infection in hospitals and in contacts with patients. Dromedary flu is endemic among young camels in Saudi Arabia. They separate corona viruses from their noses and sometimes in the stool. Only recently people and dromedary camels share the same corona viruses. The corona virus first adapted in the herds of camel breeders, especially in newborn camels. Young camels are more susceptible to the corona virus, because of their lower immunity status and the smoother virus replication. Dromedaries bred as dairy cattle (females) showing highest serum titers, followed by camels being bred for meat (mostly

males) and finally the dromedaries used for transport activities (also mostly males) have been found to be the least susceptible to the virus. Young camels that do not have antibodies have a high chance of becoming infected and, in turn, expose the mothers to infection or reinfection. Camels are also bred in Burkina Faso, Ethiopia and Morocco under the same conditions. Today the MERS-CoV circulates from person to person. Corona viruses adapted to humans spread through the airways and circulate more and more in society. With the annual Hajj pilgrimage to Mecca, more than 2 million Muslims, from more than 180 countries, are at risk of becoming infected with MERS-CoV and spreading. Saudi authorities warn not to drink unpasteurized camel milk and to wear gloves when caring for the animals. The omnipresence of the animals, their importance for the economy of the regions and their popularity will continue to promote the transfer of this coronavirus from dromedary to human.

Employee risks in the meat industry

An increased mortality of brain tumors has been observed in veterinary surgeons (Blair A). Veterinarians and Artificial Insemination assistants do a lot of internal examination on cows. Transmission via the uterus and the birth canal during labor, of bovine leukemia virus (BLV) plays a crucial role in spread and persistence of BLV infection in cattle (Mekata H).

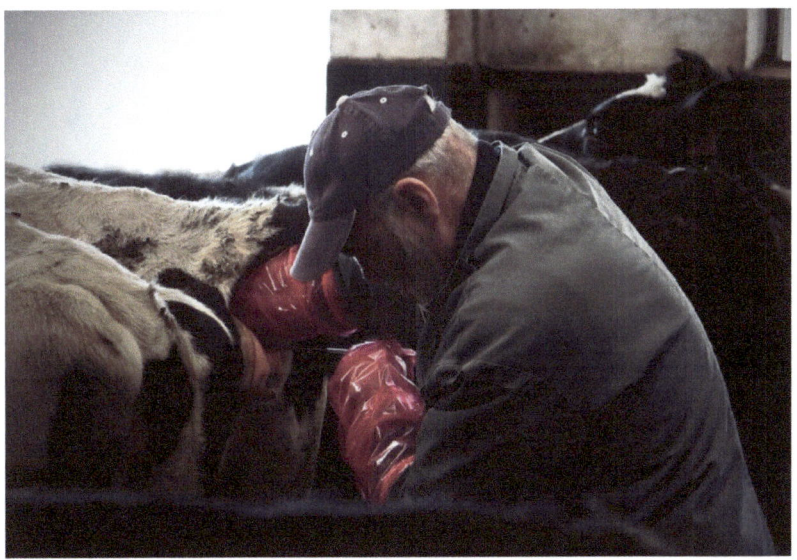

In their work, veterinarians and AI staff come into contact with bovine leukemia virus, a carcinogenic virus. Bovine leukemia is an economically important infection of dairy cattle worldwide, caused by bovine leukemia virus (BLV). The presence of infections in Canadian dairy herds is high and is still increasing. Seventy percent of the herds were identified as BLV positive (one or more positive animals).

Nekouei O, VanLeeuwen J, Sanchez J, Kelton D, Tiwari A, Keefe G Herd-level risk factors for infection with bovine leukemia virus in Canadian dairy herds. Prev Vet Med. 2015; 119 (3-4)

The deaths of 5,016 veterinarians were examined and compared with those of the general American population. The mortality rates were significantly increased from malignant lymphomas and leukemia, colon, brain and skin. Less mortality was found for stomach and lung cancer.

Blair A, Hayes HM Jr. (1982) Mortality patterns among US veterinarians, 1947-1977: an expanded study. Int J Epidemiol. 1982 Dec;11(4):391-7.

Increased risk of esophageal, colon, brain and pancreatic cancer and melanoma in veterinarians in Sweden could not be explained by the socio-economic status of this profession. Occupational exposures to carcinogenic viruses in livestock are potential sources.

Travier N, Gridley G, Blair A, Dosemeci M, Boffetta P. (2003) Cancer incidence among male Swedish veterinarians and other workers of the veterinary industry: a record-linkage study. Cancer Causes Control. 2003 (6):587-93.

Cows are constantly re-impregnated after the birth of the calves by artificial insemination, so that their milk will never stop flowing. Their calves grow up to become dairy cows or are reared for veal. For production of milk and cheese, the mother cow must give birth to as many calves as possible. Female calves grow up to become dairy cows, bulls go to the meat industry. Milk, cheese and meat production are inextricably linked. Artificial insemination (AI) in cows is not something of recent years. Artificial insemination was already introduced in Friesland in dairy cows in 1935. The sperm is frozen in "straws" and then introduced by a veterinarian or AI assistant to the animal at the right time, depending on the time of the ovulation cycle. Calves are taken away from their mother soon after birth.

Employee risks in the poultry industry

Carcinogenic viruses are found and cause tumors in chickens and turkeys. A number are carriers and diffusers of these infectious viruses. Virus has been shown in chicken products and eggs, so exposure to humans is universal and almost unavoidable. These viruses are not very contagious, but still have the ability to infect and transform human cells. Antibodies against avian leukemia sarcoma viruses (ALSV) and reticulo endothelial viruses (REV) have been found in blood sera of workers in poultry slaughterhouses. Mortality from cancer has been studied in 20,132 workers in poultry slaughterhouses and processing plants, a group with the highest human exposure to these viruses. The mortality rate among poultry workers has been compared with that of the American population as a whole. Substantially increased risks were observed in poultry workers as a whole or in subgroups, for different cancers: cancer of the mouth and pharynx; pancreas; trachea / bronchus / lung; brain; cervix; lymphocytic leukemia; monocytic leukemia; and tumors of the blood-forming and lymphatic systems. This study provides evidence that a group of people with high exposure to carcinogenic viruses, occurring in poultry, are at a higher risk of death from a number of cancers. Antibodies have been shown in the blood of these workers against avian leukemia viruses (ALV) and reticulo endothelial viruses (REV).

Metayer C, Johnson ES, Rice JC (1998) Nested case-control study of tumors of the hemopoietic and lymphatic systems among workers in the meat industry. Am J Epidemiol 147(8):727- https://www.ncbi.nlm.nih.gov/pubmed/9554414

Johnson ES, Ndetan H, Lo KM (2010) Cancer mortality in poultry slaughtering / processing plant workers belonging a union pension fund. Environ Res 110(6):588-94 https://www.ncbi.nlm.nih.gov/pubmed/20541185

Brain cancer is more common in poultry farmers involved in killing chickens. The killing of chickens was accompanied by an almost 6-fold increase in the risk of brain cancer. Chick culling is the process of killing newly hatched poultry for which the industry has no use. It occurs in all industrialized egg production whether free range, organic, or battery cage - including that of the UK and US. Because male chickens do not lay eggs and only those on breeding pro- grams are required to fertilize eggs, they are considered redundant to the egg-laying industries and are usually killed after they hatch and shortly after being sexed. Many methods of culling do not involve anesthetic and include cervical dislocation, asphyxiation by carbon dioxide and maceration using a high-speed grinder. Workers in poultry slaughterhouses and processing plants often process thousands of chickens daily, come into contact with poultry meat, organs and blood and run the risk of injuries that form a route for viruses and other microbial substances to enter the body. They also work for longer periods in confined spaces, which increases the risk of inhaling microbes. Viruses that are known to cause cancer in poultry can be responsible for the increased incidence of cancer in poultry farmers killing chickens.

Gandhi S, Felini MJ, Nidetan H, Cardarelli K, Jadhav S, Faramawi M, Johnson ES (2014) A pilot case cohort study of brain cancer in poultry and control workers. Nutr Cancer. https://www.ncbi.nlm.nih.gov/pubmed/24564367

Professor Johnson, an epidemiologist at the University of Fort Worth Texas, has published more than 30 articles in scientific journals about increased cancer risks for employees in the meat industry, many of which are specifically for poultry farmers. To definitively link the cancer risk to occupational exposure, he has developed and patented the only test to date that can detect the presence of carcinogenic viruses in the genome of tumor cells of workers with these cancers.

Brain tumors and artificial insemination of cattle

Blair A, Hayes HM Jr. (1980) Cancer and other causes of death among U.S. veterinarians, 1966-1977. Int J Cancer. 1980 Feb 15;25(2):181-5

Blair A, Hayes HM Jr. (1982) Mortality patterns among US veterinarians, 1947-1977: an expanded study. Int J Epidemiol. 1982 Dec;11(4):391-7.
https://www.ncbi.nlm.nih.gov/pubmed/7152791

Contini C, Seraceni S, Cultrera R et al. (2010) Chlamydia pneumonia Infection and Its Role in Neurological Disorders. Interdiscip Perspect Infect Dis. 2010: 273573 Section of Infectious Diseases, Department of Clinical and Experimental Medicine, University of Ferrara, Italy https://www.ncbi.nlm.nih.gov/pubmed/20182626

Gutiérrez G, Alvarez I, Merlini R, Rondelli F, Trono K Dynamics of perinatal bovine leukemia virus infection. BMC Vet Res. 2014 Apr 4;10:82.

Iwata N, Ochiai K, Hayashi K, Ohashi K, Umemura T. **Avian retrovirus infection causes naturally occurring glioma**: isolation and transmission of a virus from so-called fowl glioma. Avian Pathol. 2002 Apr;31(2):193-9.
https://www.ncbi.nlm.nih.gov/pubmed/12396365

Johnson ES 2010, Ndetan H, Lo KM Cancer mortality in poultry slaughtering / processing plant workers belonging a union pension fund. Environ Res 110:588-94
https://www.ncbi.nlm.nih.gov/pubmed/20541185

Mekata H, Sekiguchi S, Konnai S, Kirino Y, Honkawa K, Nonaka N, Horii Y, Norimine J (2015) Evaluation of the natural perinatal transmission of bovine leukaemia virus.
Vet Rec. 2015 Mar 7;176(10):254

Mekata H, Sekiguchi S, Konnai S, Kirino Y, Horii Y, Norimine J.(2015) Horizontal transmission and phylogenetic analysis of bovine leukemia virus in two districts of Miyazaki, Japan. J Vet Med Sci. 2015 Sep;77(9):1115-20

Nekouei O, VanLeeuwen J, Sanchez J, Kelton D, Tiwari A, Keefe G Herd-level risk factors for infection with bovine leukemia virus in Canadian dairy herds. Prev Vet Med. 2015 May 1;119(3-4):105-13

Travier N, Gridley G, **Blair A**, Dosemeci M, Boffetta P. (2003) Cancer incidence among male Swedish veterinarians and other workers of the veterinary industry: a record-linkage study. Cancer Causes Control. 2003 Aug;14(6):587-93.
https://www.ncbi.nlm.nih.gov/pubmed/12948290

Diseases later in life resulting from fast food

Increased consumption of energy, animal proteins, animal fats and red meat was produced in different regions of the world after the transition to a more industrialized diet, hamburgers, sugary drinks and fast food in these countries.

United States of America
Western Europe
The Netherlands
Middle East
East Asia, Japan and Korea
Polynesia

United States of America

With more than 225 million overweight people in 2016, the USA has the largest number of overweight people in the world. The USA also export these unhealthy eating habits around the world. Worse diet is the leading cause of morbidity and mortality in the United States. With an average life expectancy of 78.1 years the United States comes in only at number fifty of the world ranking list, despite being the richest nation on the planet with the most advanced medical technology. The Netherlands is slightly better with an average life expectancy of 79.2 years, less than most other European countries. Even in spite of the nation's alarming high suicide rate Japanese live 82.1 years on average.

Diseases relating to diet are the leading causes of death to the United States. The number of people overweight or obese increased between 1990 and 2016. In the most comprehensive study of US health to date, poor diet was found to be the leading cause of morbidity and mortality, even surpassing smoking. Poor diet contributed to 14 percent, while smoking accounted for 11 percent. Obesity and high blood pressure accounted for 11 and eight percent respectively.

The number one cause of death in America is the American diet. High blood pressure by fifty-five, heart attacks at sixty, maybe even cancer at seventy, and so on... For most of the leading causes of death, the science shows that the genes often account for only 10-20% of the risk at most. For example, when people move from low-risk to high-risk countries, their disease rates almost always change to those of the new environment. New diet, new diseases. But the reverse is also true. If we're eating the Standard American Diet and switch to a diet higher in whole plant foods, such as fruits and vegetables, this may lower your risk.

Western Europe

Cancer is now the most common cause of death in Western Europe, more often than chronic obstructive pulmonary disease (COPD) and cardiovascular disease and diabetes (IHD). While mortality rates for COPD and IHD are declining due to improved health care, mortality rates for cancer have increased. Our Western eating habits and addiction to animal proteins in the form of ground beef, hamburgers and all kinds of meat products are the cause of the increase in cancer. The consumption of animal fats and proteins has increased considerably since the last century. The production of meat (products), poultry, pork and other meat tripled between 1980 and 2010 and is likely to double again by 2050. At present, 70 billion farm animals are being bred annually for food. In 2050 there will be 500 million more cattle, 200 million more pigs, 1 billion more sheep and goats and 18 billion extra poultry than in 2005.
As we get older, we notice which unhealthy lifestyle habits have taken possession of us. The body constantly renews itself through the ingested diet and within a few years all cells and tissues are constantly being completely rebuilt. With age, the choice of animal or vegetable protein and fat in the daily diet is of great importance for protection against chronic diseases and cancer. Cardiovascular disease, obesity and uncontrolled growth of derailed cells are the result of an excess of animal proteins and fats in the daily diet. The chicken leukemia virus and bovine leukemia virus in our food chain are related to common cancers. The time without symptoms is 50% - 70% of the total growth of a tumor and cancer usually reveals itself at a later age.

The Netherlands

Country	Cigarette packs of 20 per year in 1970	Lung cancer mortality per 100,000 men in 1984 (CBS NL)	per 100.000 men in 2010 (EUROSTAT)
Italy	84	77	73
Norway	88	43	71
France	92	65	87
Finland	93	87	73
The Netherlands	**108**	**117**	**108**
Belgium	**119**	**119**	**115**
West Germany	125	73	West & East Germany 79
Japan	*141*	*43*	
United Kingdom	**153**	**100**	**82**
USA	*184*	*84*	

Age standardized lung cancer mortality (ICD 162 per 100,000 men per year) in ten different countries in 1984, 2007 and 2010 in relation to per adult consumption of manufactured / hand-rolled cigarettes in 1970.

In 2012, cancer was the cause of 31% of all deaths in the Netherlands (Eurostat). Today about half of all men and one third of all women develop cancer and about 20% of all deaths are due to cancer. This is an impressive increase and seems to show that the increase in cancer is a recent biological event.

- Most lung cancer in the Netherlands, Belgium and the United Kingdom. These three countries have the largest share in the international trade and import of tropical birds via Amsterdam Schiphol, Brussels Zaventhem and London Heathrow respectively.
- In Japan and the USA (see the table) there has always been a lot more smoking and the mortality rates of lung cancer were much lower.

Mortality from breast and prostate cancer is also very high compared to other countries. According to the World Health Organization, since 1980 the Netherlands has had the lowest growth in life expectancy at the birth of a total of seventeen EU countries. With regard to life expectancy for the entire population, we also score low. The mortality rate among the elderly is remarkably high. Cancer has been the number one cause of death in the Netherlands for a number of years. In seventeen European countries, our country with the mortality from cancer is in 13th place, almost at the bottom of the ranking. Child mortality in the first year of life in 15th place.

The Netherlands traditionally has a lot of animal husbandry. The poultry chain in the Netherlands consists of breeding farms, hatcheries, slaughterhouses and a large number of processing companies. Every year 40 million male chicks are killed on the first day because there is no destination for them in meat production. The Netherlands is the number 2 in the world in terms of exports of agricultural products. There is overproduction of calves, piglets, chicks, eggs, dairy products and meat products. In 2016, the record amount was more than 88 billion euros. Calf mortality is relatively high in the Netherlands and is increasing every year. The priority is too much with the cows. Only 30 percent of the calves become a dairy cow. The rest is sold to veal calves and is a residual product.

Recently published research has shown that the Netherlands has the best healthcare in the world. The government has measured this by cost-effective analyzes and research into patient satisfaction. Unfortunately, the Dutch do not have the best health. Mortality for the age of 60 and the number of chronic illnesses among the elderly have not been taken into account. The consumption of animal fats and proteins has increased considerably. Fruits and vegetables are eaten too little. An increase in diseases that pass from animals to humans is the result of the consumption of meat, animal fats and eggs from the supermarket, and the breeding of tropical birds as a hobby. Cardiovascular diseases and the unrestrained growth of derailed cells are the result of this.

- Intensive breeding of pigs, poultry, cattle and fish has become the new business model in the middle of the 20th century. All meat is only produced with artificial insemination of the animals.
- Increase in cancer is, very recently, since the middle of the 20th century.
- Carcinogenic viruses such as chicken and bovine leukemia viruses are now found in our food chain with more sophisticated laboratory research.
- Bovine leukemia virus has been shown in women's breast tissue.
- Red meat consumption is a proven risk for colon cancer.

- In the last 50 years, our diet has become increasingly unnatural. Meat, milk and eggs in our diet contribute more to climate change in the world than the emissions from our fleet. The fast-growing meat industry produces more greenhouse gases than all traffic combined.
- Fatter beef, chicken meat and pork contain more animal proteins and saturated animal fats and lead to more affluent diseases such as cardiovascular diseases, strokes, obesity and breast and colon cancer.
- Repeated bird flu infections with Chlamydia pneumonia in bird breeders increase the risk of lung cancer and malignant lymphomas.

Middle East

In 2013, when I flew over the Arabian Peninsula, I saw the integrated crop circles of Saudi Arabia. Saudi farmers feed the production of grains in the desert by winning underground water supplies. Part of that water dates back 20,000 years, until the last ice age, when more moderate conditions filled aquifers. On the ground these circles are as wide as the water-bearing layers deep, about one kilometer. Sprinklers with central pivotal pits draw from the groundwater. Many of the crops are grown to feed the intensive livestock industry. Camels are rarely used as a means of transport. Dromedary camels are bred for their milk and meat and to participate in camel races. The Saudi kingdom has implemented a multi-faceted program to supply large quantities of water, necessary to realize the spectacular growth of the agricultural sector. Expansive underground waterreservoirs have been drained through deep wells. So the desert was transformed into fertile farmland.

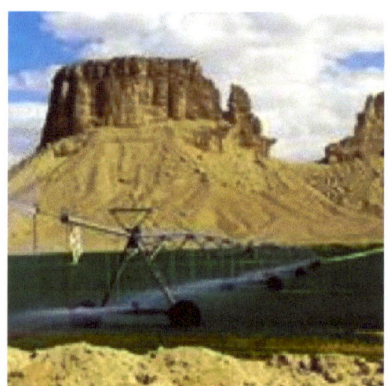

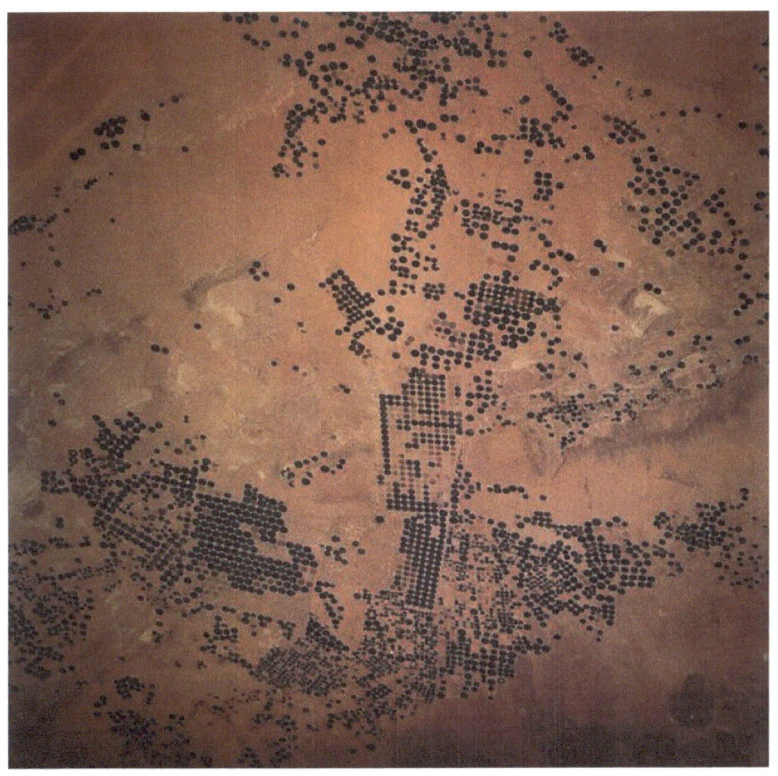

Crop circles on the Arab peninsula

Dromedary flu, from virus-spreading young camels, is the result of intensive camel breeding on the Arab peninsula. There is a rapid increase in the number of reported infections with Middle East Respiratory Syndrome Corona Virus (MERS-CoV). Since June 2012, MERS-CoV has infected more than 1,814 people, with 734 deaths (41%). The disease first occurred on the Arabian Peninsula, in Saudi Arabia and the United Arab Emirates. Concerns about the situation have increased considerably, particularly concerns about the spread of the infection in hospitals and in contacts with patients. Dromedary camel flu is endemic among young dromedary camels in Saudi Arabia. Sick dromedary camels separate corona viruses from their noses and sometimes in feces. Only recently people and dromedary camels share the same corona viruses. The corona virus first adapted in the herds of camel breeders, with larger concentrations of young dromedary camels. The breeding and weaning season is a factor. Young camels are more susceptible to camel flu because of their lower immunity status and they promote virus amplification. Today the MERS-CoV circulates from person to person and is less virulent. These humanized corona viruses pass through the airways and are increasingly common in society. Without stopping the transmission of these camels flu, we will continue to see more human cases in the Middle East. With the annual Hajj Pilgrimage to Mecca in October, more than 2 million Muslims from more than 180 countries are at risk of receiving MERS-CoV and spreading it to their home countries. Saudi authorities warn their citizens against drinking unpasteurized camel milk and advise them to wear gloves when they care for the animals. The omnipresence of the animals, their importance for the economy of the region and their popularity mean that the transfer of MERS-CoV to the camels to humans will continue to take place. The father of the current Syrian president promised his people full granaries and more meat pots. In Syria too, water sources were tapped to promote agriculture and livestock farming. A drought period and shortages of water drove the farming population en masse to the cities. Great social unrest ensued. The popular uprising in Syria is brutally precipitated. Poverty, war, hunger, higher temperatures, drought and lack of water mean that more and more people are fleeing from the Middle East and Central Africa.

Far East, Japan and Korea

In Japan and Korea, large-scale imports of beef and pork began after the Second World War, respectively after the Korean War. In 1970 in Japan and 1990 in Korea a sharp increase in the numbers of colon cancer was observed. Consumption of fried beef (eg shabu-shabu, Korean yukhoe and Japanese yukke) became very popular in both countries. A specific meat factor, presumably one or more thermo-resistant potential carcinogenic bovine viruses (for example polyoma, papilloma or single-stranded DNA viruses), can contaminate the beef and lead to latent infections in the intestinal tract.

zur Hausen H (2012) Red meat consumption and cancer: reasons for suspect involvement or bovine infectious factors in colorectal cancer. Int J Cancer. 2012 Jun 1; 130 (11): 2475-83
https://www.ncbi.nlm.nih.gov/pubmed/22212999

Increased consumption of energy, animal fat and Red meat has occurred in East Asia in recent decades. Data on breast cancer, colon, prostate, esophagus and stomach cancer mortality rates for China (1988-2000), Hong Kong (1960-2006), Japan (1950-2006), Korea (1985-2006) and Singapore (1963- 2006) were obtained from the WHO. In the selected countries (except breast cancer in Hong Kong), a noticeable increase in mortality rates of breast, colon and prostate cancer and a decreasing decrease in esophageal and gastric cancer in the study periods were observed. For example, the annual percentage increase in mortality in breast cancer was 5.5% for the period 1985-1993 in Korea and the mortality rates for prostate cancer increased from 1958 to 1993 in Japan by 3.2% per year. These changes in cancer mortality followed ~ 10 years after the transition to more industrially prepared food, hamburgers, sugary drinks and fast food in these countries.

Zhang J, Dhakai IB, Zhao Z, Li L (2012) Trends in mortality from cancers of the breast, colon, prostate, esophagus, and stomach in East Asia: role of nutrition transition. Eur J Cancer Prev 2012 Sep; 21 (5): 480-9
https://www.ncbi.nlm.nih.gov/pubmed/22357483

Mortality rates for prostate cancer have increased dramatically (25x) in Japan after the Second World War. After the war the consumption of milk increased by 20x, from meat 9x and from eggs 7x. Milk contains large amounts of estrogens plus proteins and saturated fats. The recent increase in its use is likely to be the cause of the surge of prostate cancer in Japan.

Ganmaa D, Li XM, Qin LQ et al. The experience of Japan as a clue to the etiology of testicular and prostatic cancers. Med Hypotheses. 2003 May; 60 (5): 724-30
https://www.ncbi.nlm.nih.gov/pubmed/12710911

Polynesia

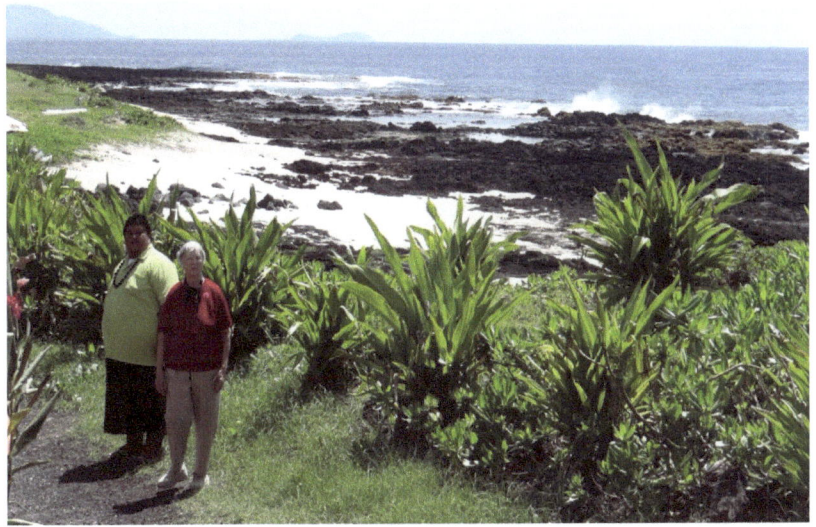

The inhabitants of Tuvalu, Fiji, Samoa and the Cook Islands are massively overweight. According to the World Health Organization (WHO), nine of the world's ten thickest countries belong to the Pacific Islands. Tonga (4th, 90.8%), Samoa (6th, 80.4%) and USA (9th, 74.1%). Up to 95 percent of the adult population is overweight in some countries. The number of people with obesity, extremely overweight, varies from 35 to 50 percent. The Cook Islands (90.9% overweight) are in third place in the world ranking. Slightly more than half of the population suffers from obesity. Inexpensive factory processed food has replaced the original diet of fresh fish and vegetables. Fresh fish is relatively expensive, with this money you can buy multiple hamburger meals. A bottle of cola is cheaper here than a bottle of water. 75% of the women on Samoa are extremely overweight.
https://youtu.be/RSwpX15ZNcA

Dairy Industry

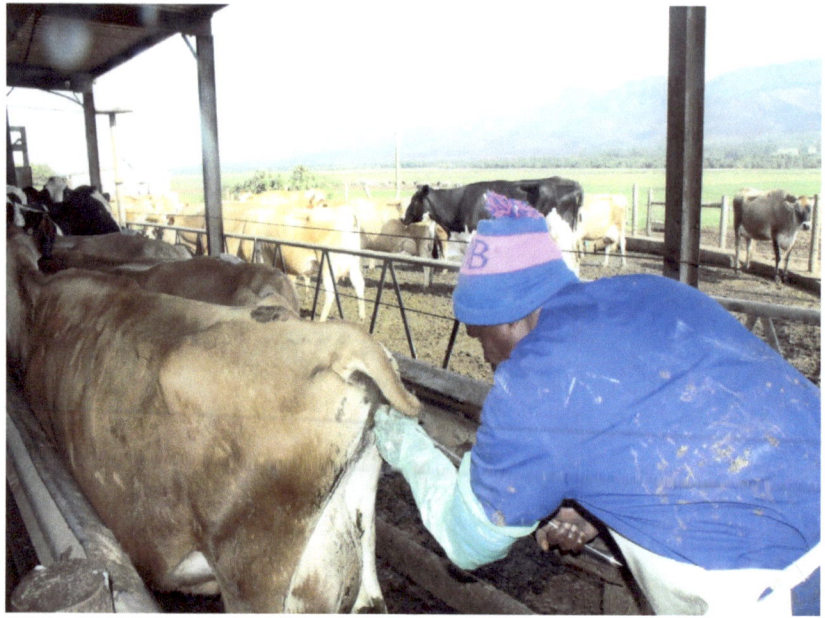

Cows are constantly re-impregnated after the birth of the calves by artificial insemination, so that their milk will never stop flowing. Their calves grow up to become dairy cows or are reared for veal. For production of milk and cheese, the mother cow must give birth to as many calves as possible. Female calves grow up to become dairy cows, bulls go to the meat industry. Milk, cheese and meat production are inextricably linked.

Raw Egg Proteins and raw milk products

Insufficient heating of chicken egg proteins
Industrially processed food contains a large proportion of liquid chicken egg proteins that in some cases are not sufficiently heated processed. Eggs are released on crushers, egg yolk and white are separated, eggshells and hail cords are removed by filters and the protein product is heated to 56 ° Celsius. In the Netherlands (1983), 20,000 tons of liquid chicken protein was produced for the industry, which was marginally pasteurized sometimes insufficiently heat treated. The confectioner processes a large number of products that contain eggs. This can be the pasteurized proteins, or he processes fresh eggs. The "whites" are collected in a special container. Housewives also sometimes come into contact with raw egg proteins when making cake batter or desserts at home. Or if they whip up the raw egg proteins.

Raw egg proteins are processed in:
SUGAR GLAZE raw egg whites with powdered sugar
ROOM FONDANT raw egg whites with butter, sugar and liqueur
OMELET SIBÉRIEN raw egg whites with sugar
BAVAROIS raw egg whites with sugar, cream, gelatin, fruits
ICE CREAM raw egg whites with sugar, milk and cream.

And also in:
STEAK TARTAR with a raw egg

Raw milk products
Raw milk is milk from cows, sheep, or goats that has not been pasteurized to kill harmful bacteria. This raw, unpasteurized milk can carry dangerous bacteria such as Salmonella, E. coli and Listeria, which are responsible for causing numerous foodborne illnesses. These harmful

bacteria can seriously affect the health of anyone who drinks raw milk, or eats foods made from raw milk. However, the bacteria in raw milk can be especially dangerous to people with weakened immune systems, older adults, pregnant women, and children.

Pasteurization is a process that kills harmful bacteria by heating milk to a specific temperature for a set period of time; 1st developed by Louis Pasteur in 1864, pasteurization kills harmful organisms responsible for such diseases as listeriosis, typhoid fever, tuberculosis, diphtheria, and brucellosis. While pasteurization has helped provide safe, nutrient-rich milk and cheese for over 120 years, some people continue to believe that pasteurization harms milk and that raw milk is a safe, healthier alternative.

Common myths and proven facts about milk and pasteurization:
- Pasteurizing milk DOES NOT cause lactose intolerance and allergic reactions. Both raw milk and pasteurized milk can cause allergic reactions in people sensitive to milk proteins.
- Raw milk DOES NOT kill dangerous pathogens by itself.
- Pasteurization DOES NOT reduce milk's nutritional value.
- Pasteurization DOES NOT mean that it is safe to leave milk out of the refrigerator for extended time, particularly after it has been opened.
- Pasteurization DOES kill harmful bacteria.
- Pasteurization DOES saves lives.

Why people have become carnivores

The slaughtering of animals is a result of our ancestors' struggle against wild animals, lions, elephants, bears etc.

From Africa and the Middle East, homo sapiens reached Western Europe 45,000 years ago.

- In that period, lions and other predators were still in the majority
- Neanderthals were the first to make the art of fire in Europe
- With wooden arrows and stone axes, there was control over lions, bears and other wild predators
- Modern man has gotten smaller jaws and larger brain contents than the Neanderthals by cooking and roasting meat

In the Colosseum, fighting of humans against wild animals took place until the 6th century. In bullfights, such as in modern corridas, bulls were hunted by helpers until they became angry: the toreros, the real hunters, fought the bull on foot, with a club or a lance. Other bullfights were related to skills similar to those depicted on famous Cretan photographs or contemporary rodeos: unarmed men on horseback rode on the bull to defeat him and then jumped on the bull to throw him down and turn his neck.

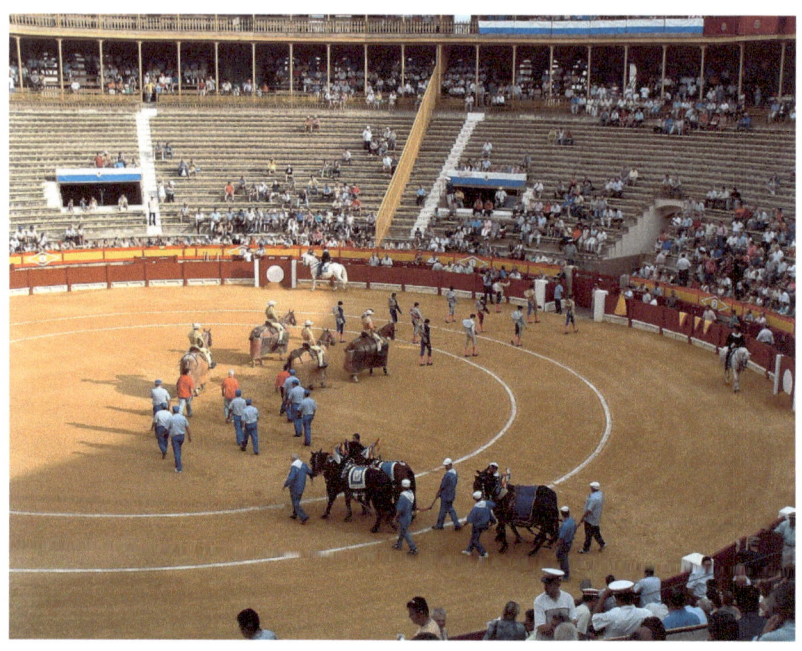

Parade of a bullfight (Plaza de Toros, Alicante)

- Bullfighters walk in front

- The helpers follow

- Picadores on horseback

- Animal handlers

- Cleanup team for killed bulls

- Butchers close the procession

Fishmeal industry

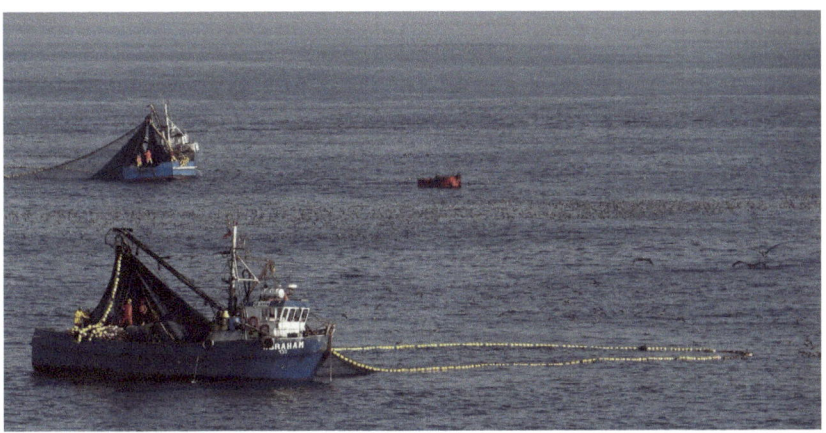

Anchovy from the southeast of the Pacific Ocean is sold as cattle feed to Europe's factory farms. Approximately one third of the total catch is fed to consumption animals, mostly farmed fish, pigs and chickens. European fishermen are obliged to land all by-catches by 2020. In addition to the by-catches, the fish-processing industry also produces a significant amount of reusable waste, such as skins, bones, fish heads and internal organs. Fish meal can be created by hydrolysis of the fish from the by-catches and fish remains, which is a great need. Especially at the fish farms in the Mediterranean. Tuna, salmon, cattle, pigs and chickens grow faster and fatter by fishmeal. More profit can be achieved and the time to slaughter is shortened. For production of fish oil and fishmeal, some 20-30 million tons of fish, anchovies, herring, mackerel and sprat species have been removed from the southeastern Pacific Ocean over the past decades. Consumption on a large scale of small glass eels, and of caviar, fish eggs, is also harmful to fish stocks.

Going back 1000 years in Europe, it was declines in freshwater fish thanks to human pressure which first pushed fishermen out into the oceans in larger numbers. Five hundred years ago, it was the decline of coastal fish that brought deep-sea trawling into existence. A hundred and fifty years ago there was still enough room on the planet. The population growth was still within the carrying capacity of the planet. Today, with the inhabitants of China or India alone equal to those of the entire planet in 1850, humanity has expanded to the point where we are crashing. The earth is overpopulated. As with agriculture, it is not the small businesses that consume the most aid, they are the industrial producers. Worldwide 20 billion is awarded annually. 6.3 billion is spent on subsidies for fuel alone; an extra 8 billion goes to the maintenance of the major ports. Small fishing uses 75% less energy to catch the same volume of fish, more environmentally friendly and with many more people. Abolish these subsidies and industrial fishing suddenly becomes a much less profitable business.

Mega farms with only cows, calves, pigs or chickens feed the animals with soy flour, fish meal and low doses of antibiotics to fatten the animals faster and to gain more profit. This has drastically increased the animal fat content of steak, pork and chicken meat. Welfare diseases such as cardiovascular diseases, increased blood pressure, excess weight and diabetes increase due to food with a high content of saturated animal fat.

Bowel Cancer

An increased risk of colorectal cancer has long been shown for the consumption of undercooked red meat. Fish and chicken do not increase this risk, although comparable or even higher concentrations of potentially cancer-causing chemicals are released during roasting or frying. In Japan and Korea, beef and pork were imported on a large scale after the Second World War and the Korean War. A strong increase in the number of patients with colon cancer was observed after 1970 in Japan and after 1990 in Korea. The consumption of undercooked beef (eg, Shabu-shabu, Korean Yukhoe and Japanese Yukke) became very popular in both countries.

Bovine leukemia virus as a source of colon cancer
A specific beef factor, probably one or more heat-resistant carcinogenic bovine viruses (for example, polyoma, papilloma or bovine leukemia virus BLV) can infect the beef and cause latent and persistent intestinal infections after human consumption (Zur Hausen H).

Polyoma viruses in hamburgers
In chopped beef samples three types of polyoma virus have been shown, which are resistant to BBQ temperatures and are carcinogenic to their natural hosts. Animal viruses are frequently found in meat products and can cause colon cancer in humans. The papilloma and polyoma viruses in particular are resistant to medium-heated steak tartar, in which the central parts of the meat are not heated above 40 - 70 degrees Celsius. These viruses endure 80 degrees Celsius for 30 minutes without losing too much of their ability to cause infections. These viruses are also insufficiently inactivated during the pasteurization of dairy products.

Acid-resistant bacteria and stomach cancer

Two Australian GPs realized that mycobacteria (acid-solid organisms) can survive the acidic environment of the stomach, which other pathogenic bacteria cannot. They discovered one of the most important human pathogens, Helicobacter pylori, which are capable of causing severe stomach inflammatory disease. It was then discovered that these microbes cause gastric carcinoma.

References bowel cancer

Hirsch D, Barker N, McNeil N, Hu Y, Camps J, McKinnon K, Clevers H, Ried T, Gaiser T. (2013) LGR5 positivity defines stem-like cells in colorectal cancer. Carcinogenesis. Dec 22.

Huang J, Magnusson M, Törner A, Ye W, Duberg AS (2013) Risk of pancreatic cancer among individuals with hepatitis C or hepatitis B virus infection: a nationwide study in Sweden. Br J Cancer. Oct 31. doi: 10.1038/bjc.2013.689

Lichtman MA A Bacterial Cause of Cancer: An Historical Essay. Oncologist. 2017 May;22(5):542-548

https://www.ncbi.nlm.nih.gov/pubmed/28432224

Peretti A, FitzGerald PC, Bliskovsky V, Buck CB, Pastrana DV. Hamburger polyomaviruses. J Gen Virol 2015 Apr;96(Pt 4):833-9
https://www.ncbi.nlm.nih.gov/pubmed/25568187

Takahashi H, Ishii H, Nishida N et al. (2011) Significance of cancer **stem cells** in the colon and rectum. Ann Surg Oncol. 2011 Apr;18(4):1166-74.

Xu JH, Fu JJ, Wang XL, Zhu JY, Ye XH, Chen SD (2013) Hepatitis B or C viral infection and risk of pancreatic cancer: A meta-analysis of observational studies. World J Gastroenterol. Jul 14;19(26):4234-4

Zhang J, Dhakai IB, Zhao Z, Li L (2012) Trends in mortality from cancers of the breast, colon, prostate, oesophagus, and stomach in East Asia: role of nutrition transition. Eur J Cancer Prev 2012 Sep;21(5):480-9
https://www.ncbi.nlm.nih.gov/pubmed/22357483

Zur Hausen H (2012) Red meat consumption and cancer: reasons to suspect involvement of bovine infectious factors in colorectal cancer. Int J Cancer.130(11):2475-83
https://www.ncbi.nlm.nih.gov/pubmed/22212999

Breast Cancer

People are exposed to carcinogenic viruses that often occur in animals in the food chain, such as laying hens, eggs, broiler chickens and dairy cows. The Avian Leukemia Virus (ALV) and Bovine Leukemia Viruses (BLV) are RNA viruses and have been shown in breast cancer cells.

Bovine Leukemia Virus in breast cancer cells

Breast cancer and ovarian cancer were rare in Japan, compared with other countries. The mortality rates, however, are increasing. After the Second World War changes in lifestyle took place in Japan. In the past 50 years (1947-1997), mortality rates of breast and ovarian cancer increased 2- and 4 fold, and the respective intake of milk, meat and eggs increased 20, 10 and 7-fold. The increase in death rates from breast cancer and ovarian cancer could be attributed to the increased consumption of animal nutrition, which occurred after 1945. Milk, dairy products and eggs are probably the cause of this (Buehring). Cows are often infected with bovine leukemia virus (BLV), a carcinogenic virus that can be transferred from the cow to the calf via the milk or during birth. Most infected cattle seem healthy and the infection is persistent. Consumption of non-pasteurized dairy products, or cheese made from raw milk, or insufficiently heated beef at the BBQ can transmit this infectious virus to humans. About 38% of the cattle, 84% of the dairy herd, and 100% of factory farm herds in the US are infected with BLV. Less than 5% of these cattle get leukemia. With this condition the animals are not admitted to the US consumer market. The BLV virus circulates with the white blood cells through the blood of infected cattle. The BLV virus also infects the mammary gland cells of the cows and infected cells are found in cow's milk (Lanou AJ). Pasteurization of cow's milk makes the BLV ineffective.

Buehring GC (2015) has shown that 39% of people in a San Francisco Bay Area have antibodies against BLV in the blood, which is an indication of exposure to BLV. Almost all cow's milk contains BLV bovine leukemia virus. In a study of 213 women, BLV-related DNA was found in breast tissue of women with a diagnosis of breast cancer, not in breast tissue of women without history of breast cancer (Buehring).

Ovarian and fallopian tube cancer in laying hens

Ovarian cancer often occurs in laying hens (Frederickson TN). For this reason, they are usually slaughtered after the first leg year. In poultry farms, laying hens do not become older than 24 months. Avian Leukemia Virus (leucosis) is a retrovirus that infects large parts of the modern poultry farms and caused a lot of economic damage. The virus is present in chickens and eggs. Man is exposed to this. RNA viruses are single-stranded proteins that do not accurately divide. When RNA viruses divide within a host cell, they make many copies that differ from the original. Some of these copy differences increase their genetic variation and survival chances in the host. Therefore, although it is often possible to prevent a DNA virus infection with a sustainable vaccine, it is very difficult, if not impossible, to make a sustainable vaccine for an RNA virus. This also makes RNA viruses very difficult to treat with medicines.

Mice also infect the grain stocks with a virus that is closely related to breast cancer viruses (Stewart TH). Free-range chickens are often kept outside, so that the risk of contamination due to the contamination of food on the ground by mouse droppings is greater. In the winter months, mice often go to poultry farms to look for food. Virus spreading mice; contamination of cereals, chicken feeds and poultry; transfer by infected chickens from viruses to the eggs; processing of raw, insufficiently heated protein in confectionery products; this is how the ALV virus arrives in humans (Pham TD).

Raw proteins often contain the ALV virus

The numbers of breast cancer that occur in humans vary geographically. No environmental factor has been able to explain this variation. The highest incidence of breast cancer worldwide occurs in countries where Mus domesticus is the native or imported type of house mouse. Stewart TH, Sage RD, Stewart AF, Cameron DW (2000) Breast cancer incidence highest in the range of one species of house mouse, Mus domesticus. Br J Cancer. 82(2):446-51.
https://www.ncbi.nlm.nih.gov/pubmed/10646903

Breast and colon cancer are not caused by breathing bad air. A causal relationship will be found earlier for pathogens in our diet. Animal proteins in milk and dairy products, in meat products and in egg proteins carry carcinogenic viruses. Improved laboratory techniques provide increasing evidence. Here is a study that makes you think.
Ji J, Sundquist J, Sundquist K Lactose intolerance and reduced risk of lung, breast and ovarian cancers: aetiological clues from a population-based study in Sweden. Br J Cancer. 2015 Jan 6; 112 (1): 149-52
https://www.ncbi.nlm.nih.gov/pubmed/25314053

A total of 22,788 persons with lactose intolerance were examined, who did not use milk products, and compared with people who did use milk products. The risk of lung, breast and colon cancer appeared to be significantly reduced in the group that did not use milk products. The risk of lung, breast and colon cancer appeared to be significantly reduced in the group that did not use milk products.

Breast cancer and ovarian cancer are they ZOONOSES?

The observation that chickens may be infected with a closely related form of mouse breast cancer virus (MMTV) may be of epidemiological significance for human breast cancer. Chickens and eggs can be infected by mice and in turn pass the virus on to people. The successful infection of human cells by MMTV has already been demonstrated (Indik S 2007). MMTV can infect human cell cultures and this finding provides a possible explanation for the discovery of MMTV in patients with breast cancer. The numbers of breast cancer that occur in humans vary geographically. No environmental factor could explain this variation. The highest incidence of breast cancer worldwide occurs in countries where Mus domesticus is the native or imported type of house mouse (Stewart TH 2000).

Breast stem cells

Women who have remained childless have immature mammary cells with stem cell activity. When these cells become infected with carcinogenic virus, this infection leads to uncontrolled cell division. In the twentieth century, breast cancer was also called "nuns disease." Full-term pregnancies reduce the risk of breast cancer and the higher the number of pregnancies, the greater this protection. The risk of breast cancer decreases by 7% after every full-term pregnancy. Women who have given birth to children have a 30% lower risk than childless women. Stem cells in the mammary gland are only developed after the first full-term pregnancy. Then 80% of the stem cells mature into milk producing gland cells. The last 20% of the stem cells develop into milk-producing cells after 7 pregnancies. Immature gland cells possess stem cell properties. The stem cell properties cause uncontrolled cell division at the time of infection or other forms of cell damage. The presence of breast cancer in the woman is closely related to her age. Breast cancer is most common in childless women and women around menopause. The biological regression of women begins around the time of menopause and is accompanied by a reduction of immune function of body cells. Reduced cell defenses can lead to the proliferation of infected mammary cells.

References breast cancer and leukemia viruses

Buehring GC, Shen HM, Jensen HM, Choi KY, Sun D, Nuovo G. Bovine leukemia virus DNA in human breast tissue. Emerg Infect Dis 2014; 20:772–782
https://www.ncbi.nlm.nih.gov/pubmed/24750974

Buehring GC, Shen HM, Jensen HM, Jin DL, Hudes M, Block G (2015) Exposure to Bovine Leukemia Virus Is Associated with Breast Cancer: A Case-Control Study. PLoS One. 2015 Sep 2;10(9):e0134304
https://www.ncbi.nlm.nih.gov/pubmed/26332838

Frederickson TN (1987) Ovarian tumors of the hen. Environ Health Perspect 73: 35

Ganmaa D, Li XM, Qin LQ et al. The experience of Japan as a clue to the etiology of testicular and prostatic cancers. Med Hypotheses. 2003 May;60(5):724-30

Guérin M, Barrois M, Terrier MJ et al. (1988) Overexpression of either c-myc or c-erbB proto-oncogenes in human breast carcinomas: correlation with poor prognosis. Oncogene Res 3:21-31

Indik S, Günzburg WH, Salmons B, Rouault F (2005) Mouse mammary tumor virus infects human cells. Cancer Research 1;65(15):6651-9

Indik S, Günzburg WH, Kulich P, Salmons B and Rouault F (2007) Rapid spread of mouse mammary tumor virus in cultured human breast cells. Retrovirology 11;4:73
https://www.ncbi.nlm.nih.gov/pubmed/17931409

Johnson ES (1994) Poultry oncogenic retroviruses and humans. Cancer Detect Prev 18(1):9-30

Johnson PA, Giles JR (2013) The hen as model of ovarian cancer. Nat Rev Cancer 13(6):432-6

Kettmann R, Portetelle D, Mammerickx M et al. (1976) Bovine leukemia virus: an exogenous RNA oncogenic virus. Proc Natl Acad Sci U S A. 1976 Apr;73(4):1014-8

Kwon OJ, Zhang L, Ittmann MM, Xin L (2013) Prostatic inflammation enhances basal-to-luminal differentiation and accelerates initiation of prostate cancer with a basal cell origin. Proc Natl Acad Sci U S A. 2013 Dec 23

Lanou AJ (2009) Should dairy be recommended as part of a healthy vegetarian diet? Counterpoint. Am J Clin Nutr. May;89(5):1638S-1642S

Lawson JS, Heng B (2010) Viruses and Breast Cancer. Review. Cancers 2010,2,752-772

Li XM, **Ganmaa D**, Sato A (2003) The experience of Japan as a clue to the etiology of breast and ovarian cancers: relationship between death from both malignancies and dietary practices. Med Hypotheses. 2003 Feb;60(2):268-75.

Luo J, Yin X, Ma T, Lu J (2010) **Stem cells** in normal mammary gland and breast cancer. Am J Med Sci. 2010 Apr;339(4):366-70

Mehta K, Pantazis P, McQueen T, Aggarwal BB Antiproliferative effect curcumin against human breast tumor cell lines. Anticancer Drugs (1997) 8(5);470-81

Pham TD, Spencer JL, **Johnson ES** (1999). Detection of avian leukosis virus in albumen of chicken eggs using reverse transcription polymerase chain reaction. J Virol Methods 78:1-11
https://www.ncbi.nlm.nih.gov/pubmed/10204692

Pogo BG, Holland JF, Levine PH (2010) Human mammary tumor virus in inflammatory breast cancer. Cancer 1;116(11):271-4
https://www.ncbi.nlm.nih.gov/pubmed/20503403

Siwko SK, Bu W, Gutierrez C, Lewis B, Jechlinger M, Schaffhausen B, Li Y Lentivirus-mediated oncogene introduction into mammary cells in vivo induces tumors. Neoplasia 2008 10(7):653-62

Stewart TH, Sage RD, Stewart AF, Cameron DW (2000) Breast cancer incidence highest in the range of one species of house mouse, Mus domesticus. Br J Cancer. 2000 Jan;82(2):446-51
https://www.ncbi.nlm.nih.gov/pubmed/10646903

Szabo S, Haislip AM, Garry RF (2005) Of mice, cats, and men: is human breast cancer a zoonosis? Microsc Res Tech. 68(3-4):197-208. Review
https://www.ncbi.nlm.nih.gov/pubmed/16276516

Venugopal K (1999) Avian leukosis virus subgroup J: a rapidly evolving group of oncogenic retroviruses. Res Vet Sci. 1999 Oct;67(2):113-9

Zhang J, Dhakai IB, Zhao Z, Li L (2012) Trends in mortality from cancers of the breast, colon, prostate, oesophagus, and stomach in East Asia: role of nutrition transition. Eur J Cancer Prev 2012 Sep;21(5):480-9
https://www.ncbi.nlm.nih.gov/pubmed/22357483

Lung Cancer

As a general practitioner I asked myself in the 1970s, why is it that so many people get prematurely ill and die before the age of 60? The search began for me after the first ten lung cancer patients I encountered. Of these, 6 were bird keepers / breeders.

Higher mortality before the age of 60 among those who kept and bred birds

During the survey period 28 deaths occurred before age 60 years, of which 19 were in men and 9 in women. There was no significant increase in death rates among those who kept dogs, cats or rodents, but there was a significant increase, in males and in both sexes, among those who kept birds. There were ten deaths in patients who had intensive contact with birds. Three cases stand out:
- The boy, who died at the age of 17 from a bone cancer in his leg, kept and bred continuously at least 100 tropical songbirds in a basement. You can imagine his risk of repeated bird flu and the occurrence of blood and bone marrow sepsis with slow persistent infection.
- One couple was examined from 1971 to 1979 after 3 years of marriage. The man had oligospermia. In 1976 the man had an aspecific lung infiltrate and from this time onwards epileptic seizures. In 1984 the man died aged 47 years from an ethmoid sinus carcinoma. No children were born (gravida 0). Before marriage the man had an aviary with a parrot and budgerigars and a dovecote. After marriage, the couple kept and bred about 15 pairs of canaries on their top floor permanently.
- Another couple was examined from 1975 to 1980 after 6 years of marriage. The man had ejaculatory impotence. In April

1980 the man, aged 32, sudden died while jogging in the dunes. Post-mortem examination showed aortic valve stenosis with calcification and signs of endocarditis. No children were born. The man kept and bred birds in his youth and had an aviary in his bedroom over his folding bed with many pairs of tropical birds. His father died from lung cancer at the age of 50 years. After the couple married, they kept a parrot, a Japanese nightingale, two budgerigars and a Mozambique.

Lung cancer patients ate less fruit and vegetables
The survey of eating habits showed that lung cancer patients took less vitamin C, fewer fruits and vegetables with their food intake. No difference in patients and controls could be demonstrated for inclusion of beta-carotene and for alcohol use. A big difference in the number of smoked cigarettes could be demonstrated.
Holst PAJ 1988, Kromhout D, Brand R Pet birds as an independent risk for lung cancer. Br Med J 297:1319-1321
https://www.ncbi.nlm.nih.gov/pmc/articles/PMC1834925/

Lung Cancer risk for men under 65 years of age was increased six-fold in those who kept birds
Both in the hospital case-control study and in the general practice survey in the Hague, lung cancer risk for men under 65 years of age was increased six-fold in those who had kept birds as pets 5 – 14 years before diagnosis of the lung cancer. This finding, coupled with the fact that one household in three or four keeps birds, implies that more than 50% of the total lung cancer rate in men under 65 years of age in The Hague can be attributed to keeping/breeding birds.

The finding of a relation between lung cancer and bird keeping/breeding for men under 65 years of age is supported by a study in West Berlin (Kohlmeier L 1992). Two studies found a relation for lung cancer patients below 55 years of age (Jöckel KH 2002, Kocazeybek B 2003). The study in Scotland (Gardiner AJ 1992) found a significant relation with pigeon keeping for patients 55-64 years of age. And the study in Taipei (Ger LP 1992) found also a significant relation between pigeon keeping and lung cancer. Anttila TI 2003, in a prospective study of Finnish women, found also a significant relation between Chlamydia pneumoniae infection and lung cancer, also among the nonsmoking women.

Younger people who breed birds are more likely to develop lung cancer
Holst PAJ Risk of lung cancer needs to be studied in younger patients who keep pet birds. BMJ (1997)
https://www.ncbi.nlm.nih.gov/pubmed/9158496
The prevalence of pet birds and of lung cancer differs between the Netherlands and Sweden. Mortality from lung cancer is much higher in the Netherlands than in Sweden—even higher than that in the United States. Compared with Sweden, the Netherlands has a higher percentage of people who breed birds and a higher concentration of the international bird trade. Breeding birds and keeping birds in family homes results in higher amounts of dust in the indoor air, poorer hygiene, and a greater risk of having infected birds. More young families than old families keep and breed household birds, and breeding is primarily a sport of adult men, not of elderly people. Cecilia Modigh and colleagues suggested (1996) that the positive results of earlier European studies could be due to the confounding influence of the higher prevalence of ownership of pet birds among the lower socio-economic classes, who have higher rates of lung cancer. This does not apply to our study in the Netherlands, which adjusted for social class. There was an important difference in the patients selected for analysis between our study in the Netherlands and the studies in Sweden and the United. Modigh and colleagues analyzed patients of all ages and have

not published an analysis of patients aged 65 and under. Our patients were aged 65 and under. During the 10 years of the general practice survey I observed that the percentage of people who kept birds seemed not to be increased among patients with lung cancer aged over 65 in my own and in colleague general practices. Younger people more often breed large amounts of tropical birds or pigeons. Elderly people often have a medical contraindication to keeping pets, having previously had lung disease. Moreover, we thought that the influence of variables other than smoking would be easier to see in younger patients, who have not had so much time to accumulate the effects of smoking over large numbers of pack years. Our study among new patients with lung cancer was designed to analyze only patients, aged 65 and under.

Experimental induction of lung cancer

Chronic inhalation studies with cigarette smoke machines, in hamsters, dogs and monkeys showed no statistically significant increase in malignant tumors in the airways, although very long exposures and high doses of smoke were used (Coggins CR 2001). These inhalation studies were performed without concomitant infection of the airways of the laboratory animals. The tobacco industry has long cited the studies as evidence for no increase in lung cancer due to smoking. Recently (Chu DJ 2012) a lung cancer animal model was developed through repeated injection of Chlamydia pneumonia in airways of rats, with or without benzo(a)pyrene. With the combination of benzo(a)pyrene and the bacteria of tropical bird flu in the spray, 44% of the laboratory rats got lung cancer.

- **Chlamydia pneumoniae of the bird cages have proven to be an independent risk factor for lung cancer.**

The combined factors of smoking and Cp chronic infection have superimposed effects and lead to greatly increased lung cancer risk.
Chu DJ, Guo SG, Pan CF, Wang J, Du Y, Lu XF, Yu ZY (2012) An experimental model for induction of lung cancer in rats by Chlamydia pneumoniae. Asian Pac J Cancer Prev. 2012;13(6):2819-22
https://www.ncbi.nlm.nih.gov/pubmed/22938465

Favorable results of combined therapy of azithromycin with the chemotherapy on non-small cell lung cancer patients

Although new chemotherapeutic drugs have been applied constantly, their efficacy for non-small cell lung cancer (NSCLC) is still not satisfactory. In recent years, epidemiological investigations have shown that lung cancer may be induced by chronic Chlamydia pneumonia

(Cpn) infection. This study (Chu DJ 2014) of azithromycin, commonly used for the treatment of Cp infections, combined with the chemotherapeutics paclitaxe and cisplatin on stage III-IV NSCLC patients achieved favorable results in terms of side effects and overall survival.

Azithromycin, a macrolide antibiotic as well as erythromycin, prevents bacteria from growing by interfering with their protein synthesis. It binds to the bacterial ribosome, thereby inhibiting the translation of mRNA and protein synthesis.

The aforementioned examinations and treatments have been applied with favorable results by treating physicians with longer existing drugs whose patents had long expired. These experiments deserve to be copied and would greatly reduce the costs of medical treatments and could open a new treatment trail apart from the doubleblind search of the pharmaceutical industry for better and more profitable drugs. My previously suggested idea of treating lung cancer with previous infections with Chlamydiae for a long time with doxycycline (a derivative form of tetracycline) can also have a favorable result.

Co-therapy with tetracycline and azithromycin (Ferreri AJ)

Malignant lymphomas were treated with tetracycline (doxycycline) and their disappearance was similar to eradication of the Chlamydia bacteria detected in the cells (Ferreri AJ 2005). Tetracycline and macrolide (erythromycin) antibiotics have a striking therapeutic effect on Chlamydia infection. Cp infection can be controlled and prevented. Penicillin kills bacteria by preventing the bacteria from rebuilding their cell wall after division. Chlamydiae have no cell wall and, like viruses, are completely dependent on their host cells. Once in the host cell, Chlamydiae are not susceptible to penicillin. Tetracyclines prevent these cell parasites from using the metabolic processes of the host cell. Chlamydiae need these to form new proteins for growth and multiplication. Tetracycline is produced from chlortetracycline, a compound derived from Streptomyces aureofaciens. Tetracyclines are able to enter the host cells of the Chlamydiae through the pores of the cell wall. Once inside the cell, tetracycline causes inhibition of DNA and protein synthesis that these cell parasites need for their own growth and multiplication.

Does cancer start with a mutation of a cell nucleus?

The concept that cancer is a genetic disease, also infers that cancer development is irreversible because reversal of mutations back to a normal cell is extremely rare. The probability of mutating a normal cell to a cancer cell during cell division is approximate one in a million or so. If we assume the same probability for a back-mutation, the probability that a cell will become cancerous then reverse course is exceptionally low (probability is about one chance in a trillion). The assumption of the pharmaceutical industry that with surgery and radiotherapy incurable cancer only can be treated with medicines is fundamentally wrong. The pharmaceutical industry has made himself master to every facet of illness. No patient leaves the office without a prescription. The costs of cancer research and care exceed the benefits of the slight progression in cancer treatment for the last 50 years. There is a poignant shortage in education in nutritional science among cancer researchers and clinicians. Prevention is preferable to cure. The pharmaceutical industry only develops and sells medicines that make money. That is not to blame commercial companies. Well-functioning, first generation antibiotics, painkillers, antihypertensive drugs etc. are replaced by newer drugs if the patents have expired.

That the ancient Egyptians drank a lot of beer is a known fact. The Nubians (South Egypt North Sudan) could also enjoy it. In 1980, anthropologist George Armelagos and medical analyst Mark Nelson of Paratek Pharmaceuticals discovered traces of the antibiotic tetracycline in human bones from 350 - 550 AD. Tetracycline is produced by streptomyces, a bacterium that is often found on grain. When fermenting grain to make beer, streptomyces produces large amounts of the antibiotic. It is therefore not surprising that tetracycline was found in the bones of the people of that time. In more recent research on the bones, Armelagos and Nelson discovered that the bones were saturated with it. Apparently the Nubians deliberately produced the antibiotic for the treatment of diseases. Even in the bones of very young children died, the substance was found in large quantities. An indication that the beer foam was prescribed to sick children. We always assumed that the discovery of tetracycline did not take place until 1948. Streptomyces grows in a gold colony that floated on top of the beer. It is possible that this golden color also had an important meaning for the Nubians.

It would grace the pharmaceutical industry if drugs were first tested on animals that get similar tumors to humans. The budgerigar with a carcinoma and the laying hen with an ovarian carcinoma are perfect models for the oncotherapist to test medicines! These birds are fully available. It has been known since 1987 that almost half of laying hens get malignant growths (Frederickson, Johnson).

Frederickson TN (1987) Ovarian tumors of the hen. Environ Health Perspect. 1987 August; 73: 35–51.

Johnson PA, Giles JR (2013) The hen as a model of ovarian cancer. Nat Rev Cancer. 2013 Jun;13(6):432-6

Follow-up references lung cancer studies

Anttila TI, Koskela P, Leinonen M et al. (2003) Chlamydia pneumoniae Infection and the Risk of Female Early-Onset Lung Cancer. Int J Cancer:107,681-682
https://www.ncbi.nlm.nih.gov/pubmed/14520711

Bruu AL, Haukenes G, Aasen S, Grayston JT, Wang SP, Klausen OG, Myrmel H, Hasseltvedt V (1991) Chlamydia pneumoniae infections in Norway 1981-87 earlier diagnosed as ornithosis. Scand J Infect Dis 23(3):299-304

Chaturvedi AK et al. (2010) Chlamydia pneumoniae infection and risk for lung cancer. Cancer Epidemiol Biomarkers Prev 1498-1505
https://www.ncbi.nlm.nih.gov/pubmed/20501758

Chu DJ, Guo SG, Pan CF, Wang J, Du Y, Lu XF, Yu ZY (2012) An experimental model for induction of lung cancer in rats by Chlamydia pneumoniae. Asian Pac J Cancer Prev. 2012;13(6):2819-22
https://www.ncbi.nlm.nih.gov/pubmed/22938465

Chu DJ, Yao DE, Zhuang YF, Hong Y, Zhu XC, Fang ZR, Yu J and Yu ZY (2014) Azithromycin enhances the favorable results of paclitaxel and cisplatin in patients with advanced non-small cell lung cancer. Genet. Mol. Res. 13(2):2976-2805
https://www.ncbi.nlm.nih.gov/pubmed/24782093

Coggins CR (2001) A review of chronic inhalation studies with mainstream cigarette smoke, in hamsters, dogs, and nonhuman primates. Toxicol Pathol. 2001 Sep-Oct;29(5):550-7

Felini M, Preacely N, Shah N, Christopher A, Sarda V, Elfaramawi M, Sall M, Bangara S, Gandhi S, **Johnson ES** (2012) A case-cohort study of lung cancer in poultry and control workers: occupational findings. Occup Environ Med. 2012 Mar;69(3):191-7

Ferreri AJ, Dolcetti R, **Magnino** S ey al. (2007) A woman and her canary: a tale of chlamydiae and lymphomas. J Natl Cancer Inst. 2007 Sep 19;99(18):1418-9
https://www.ncbi.nlm.nih.gov/pubmed/17848672

Gardiner AJ, Forey AB, Lee PN (1992) Avian exposure and bronchiogenic carcinoma. Br Med J 305 :989-992
https://www.ncbi.nlm.nih.gov/pubmed/1458146

Ger LP, Liou SH, Shen CV, Kao SJ, Chen KT (1992) Risk factors of lung cancer.
J. Formos Med Assoc Sep; 91 Suppl 3:222-231
https://www.ncbi.nlm.nih.gov/pubmed/1362909

Holst PAJ 1997 Risk of lung cancer needs to be studied in younger patients who keep and breed pet birds. Br Med J (1997) 314, 1353

Jackson LA, Wang SF, Nazar-Stewart V, Grayston IT, Vaughan IL (2000) Association of Chlamydia pneumoniae immunoglobin A seropositivity and risk of lung cancer. Cancer Epidemiol Biomarkers Prev 9(11): 1263-1266
https://www.ncbi.nlm.nih.gov/pubmed/11097237

Johnson ES, Ndetan H, Lo KM (2010) Cancer mortality in poultry slaughtering / processing plant workers belonging a union pension fund. Environ Res 110(6):588-94
https://www.ncbi.nlm.nih.gov/pubmed/20541185

Johnson ES (2012), Choi Km. Lung cancer risk in workers in the meat and poultry industries - a review. Zoonoses Public Health 59(5):303-13
https://www.ncbi.nlm.nih.gov/pubmed/22332987

Jöckel KH, Pohlabeln H, Bromen K, Ahrens W, Jahn I (2002) Pet Birds and risk of lung cancer in North-Western Germany. Lung Cancer Jul;37(1)29-34

Kocazeybek B (2003) Chronic Chlamydophila pneumoniae infection in lung cancer, a risk factor: a case-control study. J Med Microbiol 52(8):721-6

Kohlmeier L, Arminger A, Bartolomeycik S, Bellach B, Rehm J, Thamm M (1992) Pet birds as an independent risk for lung cancer: Case-control study. Br Med J 305:986-989 https://www.ncbi.nlm.nih.gov/pubmed/1458145

Koyi H, Branden E, Gnarpe J, Gnarpe H, Arnholm B, Hillerdal G (1999) Chlamydia pneumoniae may be associated with lung cancer. Preliminary report on a seroepidemiological study. APMIS 107(9):828

Laurilla AL, Antilla T, Laara E, Bloigu A, Virtamo J, Albanes D, Leinonen M, Saikku P (1997) Serological evidence of an association between Chlamydia pneumoniae infection and lung cancer. Int J Cancer 20;74(1)1-34

Littman AJ Jackson LA, Vaughan TL (2005) Chlamydia pneumoniae and lung cancer: epidemiologic evidence. Cancer Epidemiol Biomarkers Prev. 14(4):773-8
https://www.ncbi.nlm.nih.gov/pubmed/15824142

Mather JP, Roberts PE, Pan Z et al. (2013) Isolation of cancer stem like cells from human adenosquamous carcinoma of the lung supports a monoclonal origin from a multipotential tissue stem cell. PLoS One 4;8(12)

Zhan P, Suo LJ, Qian Q, Shen XK, Qiu LX, Yu LK, Song Y (2011). Chlamydia pneumoniae infection and lung cancer risk: a meta-analysis. Eur J Cancer Mar;47(5):742-7
https://www.ncbi.nlm.nih.gov/pubmed/21194924

Trade in tropical birds and pigeons

Since the slave trade and slavery were abolished 150 years ago, international trade in tropical companion animals, international human trafficking, the arms industry and drug trafficking became the most profitable forms of trade. Worldwide, an estimated 40,000 primates, 4 million exotic birds, 640,000 reptiles and 350 million tropical fish are traded live each year. The trade in exotics is estimated at an $ 6 billion industry. Bird exhibitions and bird breeders caused an explosive growth of this popular hobby
Keeping and breeding tropical birds is a hobby of young families. The ratio of breeders to the total number of bird keepers is about 1: 6. The level of organization of the large bird breeders in the Netherlands is high due to participation in the breeding competitions. Public shows, which were held several times a year, made the hobby increasingly popular in the twentieth century. When pigeons are kept together with tropical birds, Chlamydia infections are more common.

The Netherlands is in the forefront of the presence of birds as pets (17,5 million)
The American Veterinary Medicine Association (AVMA) had 11-16 million companion birds and exotic birds in the United States in 2007. In France, 6 million companion birds were owned by households in 2010. In Belgium every bred bird must be provided with a ring with a number to which the owner can identify the breeder. In 2011 the Association Ornithologique de Belgique (AOB) registered 249 ornithological associations, authorized to identify their birds by an official ring. Pet birds are a lucrative business for pet stores and local breeders, as a single male canary is already sold for around 30 euros in Belgium and a female for about 20 euros. Prices are about the same for zebra finches and budgerigars, and 50% to 100% higher for "special"

finches such as bullfinches. Bird fairs and markets for live birds also attract many people. In addition, some species are bred because of their very high value; for example, in the case of canaries, the male and female specimens with particular genetic potential are presented in the national and international competitions for their posture (the Bossu Belge), the color (red mosaic) or for their song (Harzer). Consequently, the offspring can be sold for strongly increased prices. Baby parrots are quickly removed from the nest and, for example, with syringes fed by hobby breeders. A parrot reacts like a peewit: when eggs are taken away, she puts extra for. Growers get that way not three but six eggs per round. That saves quite a lot of money. The African Grey parrot quickly produces 700 euros. The doll, the female parrot, is literally milked and is not growing old.

Several times a year these beautiful birds are brought to shows and competitions, to exchange or sell. Exotic birds such as larger parrots, macaw or cockatoo are traded legally or illegally from Asia or South America. These birds are still high on the list of popular pets and are also richly represented in zoos and parks.

How do tropical birds and pigeons transmit diseases to humans?

From the infectious diseases transmitted by cage birds to humans, a number have been adapted so that they can pass from human to human and cause epidemics. This also infects people who do not keep or breed birds.

- Highly contagious Parrot Disease (Chlamydia psittaci), Ornithosis (Chlamydia pneumoniae) and Pneumonia (Chlamydia pneumoniae and TWAR)
- Infectious inflammatory bowel disease caused by Salmonella typhimurium
- Contagious bird flu (Influenza A (viair) Virus H5N1 - H7N9)

Breeding of tropical birds

Baby parrots are quickly removed from the nest and, for example, injected with syringes by hobby breeders. A parrot reacts like a lapwing: when the eggs are removed, she puts a few extra. In this way, breeders do not get three, but six eggs per round. That saves a lot of money. An African gray parrot soon yields € 700. The doll, the female parrot, is literally milked and does not grow old. When birds are packed together in small spaces, with insufficient food and lack of sunlight, bacteria present in small numbers get a chance. Chlamydia multiplies rapidly and is excreted in large quantities. The bacteria float out of the cages, along with down feathers, powdered manure and contaminated dust particles. People can breathe in dust particles and become ill. No government is willing to ban the breeding and selling of birds, not even to insist that these birds are kept under healthier conditions.

Pigeons sport

The Dutch Post Pigeon Organization (NPO) in Utrecht had 55,000 members in 1982, with an average of 30 carrier pigeons (100 after the breeding season). The members of the NPO have about 1 - 2 million pigeons with each other, depending on the season. Members act among themselves and with the fans of the sport in Belgium. There are almost no commercial racing pigeon dealers, unless a bird trader happens to be breeding pigeons himself. The breeding of racing pigeons has become an addiction among enthusiasts. The real pigeon keeper knows each of his birds and spends most of his free time in the loft. He places bets on the performance of his birds and can reclaim his investment many times when his bird finishes first. There is a well developed system of leg rings and time clocks.

Especially, when racing pigeons or fancy pigeons are kept with other birds, they spread all kinds of bird flu. When transporting for trade, or during day trips, which make pigeons many times a year to Belgium, France, Spain or England, the birds are sent in large baskets, where there is ample opportunity for a wide spread of contaminated excrement. Previously it was thought that imported, often illegal birds, were the main source for distribution, but many domestic birds and pigeons bred in their own country have now also become infected. In 2010, the presence of the parrot disease bacteria was investigated in 32 Belgian pigeon breeding stocks and 61 wild-flying pigeons that were caught in the city of Ghent, Belgium. In addition, the transfer of the bacteria was examined in these breeding files. Carriers were often infected, at least one of the lofts was positive in 13 of the 32 (40.6%) pigeon loft stocks. Human infection was discovered in 4 of the 32 (12.5%) pigeon fanciers. This study clearly shows the possible risk of transmission of pigeons to humans from the tropical parrot bacterium.

- Pigeon breeders often use (37.5%) antibiotics for the prevention of respiratory diseases.

In a patient-controlled study in Scottish hospitals (Gardiner AJ 1992) 143 lung cancer patients of all ages were compared with 143 controls with cardiovascular disease and 143 controls with orthopedic disorders. They found a 3.9 times increased risk of lung cancer in keeping pigeons; for the younger age group 55-64 years they found a significantly increased risk of lung cancer in connection with keeping pigeons 5.62 times more (95% CI 1.58-20). Probably there were more active pigeon breeders in the younger age group.

Indoor air pollution
Significantly increased dust levels are measured in households where birds are kept. Particulate matter with a diameter of 2.5 micron or less is the most important health risk of (indoor) air pollution. The number of particles of about 2 microns is increased in bird-keeping households. Bird keepers, and especially bird breeders, have an increased risk of infection with local damage to the tissue and allergic reactions in the lung tissue. Due to excessive mucus production, there is more drainage of alveoli in smokers than in non-smokers. As a result, the dust container and antigen load is shifted from the alveoli to the smaller air tubes in the bird keeper who smokes. The antigens reach the smallest alveoli in smaller quantities and the immune responses and inflammation occur more strongly in smaller bronchi.

- The smaller bronchi are the preferred location of lung cancer.

Both smoking and keeping birds are ultimately responsible for the poor functioning of the "lung cleaning service" and a shortage of immune proteins. The result is less protection of the lung mucosal cells against continual allergen and fine material that precipitates on the thin mucus layer of the smaller air tubes and subsequently lung cancer. It is therefore possible to see why most lung tumors develop in the smaller air tubes, at some distance from the finest alveoli, where gases and dust particles circulate at first instance. Both smoking and keeping birds at home increases the dust content of the air in the house.

- Dust particles from bird cages and tobacco smoke are potentially more harmful than the particles that occur in outside air (eg pollen grains, ash, soot particles and sand grains).

- There is every reason to pay particular attention to the bird breeders among the smokers.

Felderhof-Hoytema (1987) followed 699 school children aged 4 to 16 in The Hague. Of these children, 39.6% had birds at home. In children with one or more cage birds at home, 50.9% had symptoms of Chronic Non-Specific Lung Disease compared to 19% in children without cage birds at home. Converted, this means that 50% of the more serious forms of CNSLD, are related to the presence of cage birds at home.

- It is more obvious to measure particulate matter levels in households with birds than in classrooms.

Tobacco industry

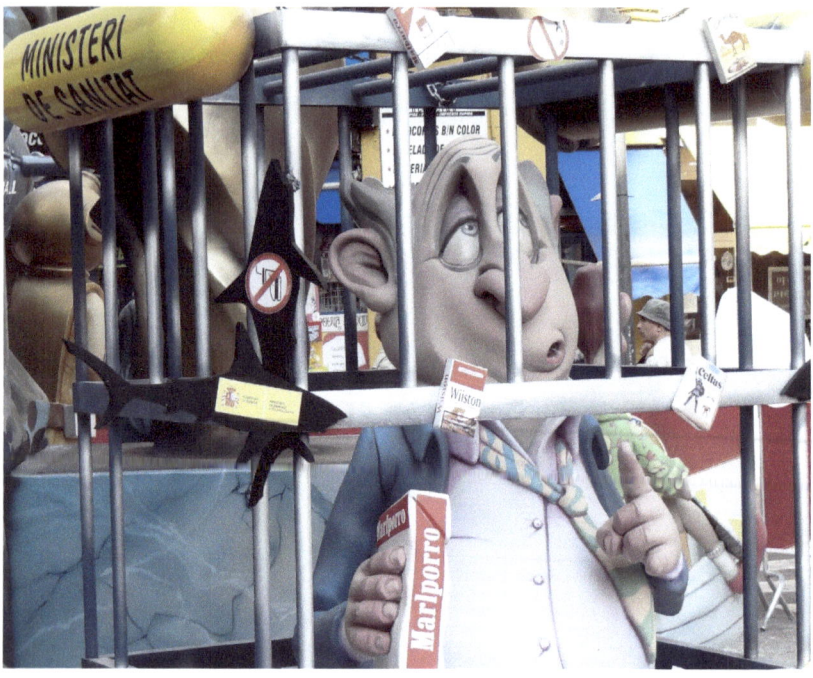

- We are all exposed to cigarette smoke and, in particular, to one of the most important carcinogenic ingredients: benzo (a) pyrene.

Smokers who breathe deep into the smoke and hold the smoke in their lungs for 2 - 3 seconds, by breathing out slowly, have a larger deposit of particles of 1 - 3 µm in their airways. The process of absorption of water vapor by hygroscopic particles in cigarette smoke is recognizable.

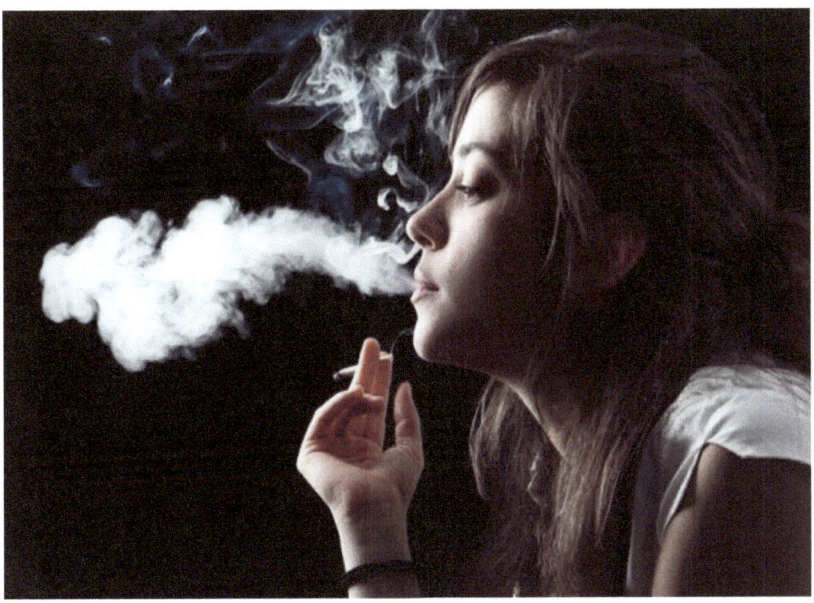

- A smoker who breathes long and deep, blows out white smoke instead of the blue smoke that is the original color of tobacco burning gases

Irritation of the respiratory tract mucous membrane as a result of smoking leads to increased mucous production. In the long run, the heavy smoker's first cigarette of the morning does not produce enough irritation to cough up all the mucus that has collected during the night. A drainage problem arises on the minute air sacs involving stasis and a diminution of the diameter of the smaller bronchi. Stasis increases the risk of infection and allergic processes if inhaled micro-organisms and antigens can reach these areas. Some smokers cough and bring up mucus. Some develop a severe bronchial obstructive syndrome, in which coughing is completed with shortness of breath and wheezing in the chest. In addition to accumulation of mucus, these patients have bronchial spasms and edema of the bronchial mucous membrane and muscles of the bronchial wall, and to allergic processes in the bronchial wall.

- Smokers who develop shortness of breath, coughs and wheezing in the chest are individuals who develop the most lung tumors.

Global warming

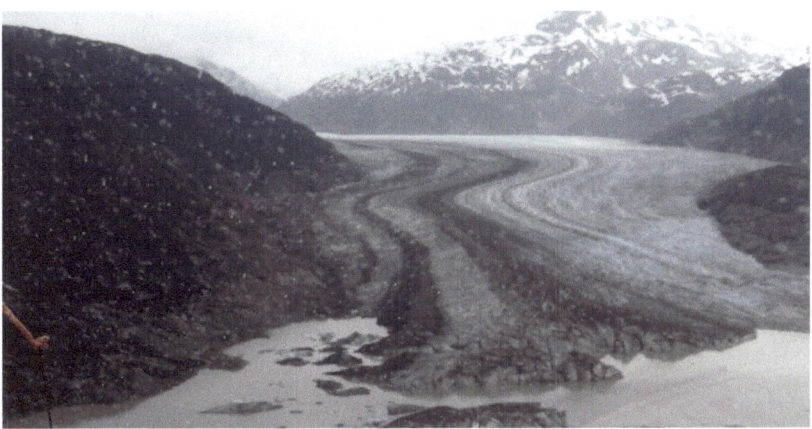

- Every year the glaciers in Alaska become hundreds of meters shorter by melting the ice. https://youtu.be/HY671_UR-qo
- In the USA, cattle emit approximately 5.5 million m3 of methane, a greenhouse gas that is 25 times more potent than CO2.

The fast-growing meat industry produces more greenhouse gases than the exhaust gases from all car traffic on earth. Melting glaciers are the result of this. Meat, milk and eggs in our food contribute more to the climate change in the world than the exhaust fumes of our fleet.
CE Delft, Fraunhofer Institute for Systems and Innovation Research and LEI Wageningen. Behavioural climate change mitigation options and their appropriate inclusion in quantitative longer-term policy scenarios. Delft, January 2012

Livestock farming accounts for at least 14.5% and, according to some studies, even 51% of man-made greenhouse gases. In the USA cattle emit approximately 5.5 million m3 of methane - a greenhouse gas that is 25 times more potent than CO2.

- All life depends on the oceans. Circulation in the North Atlantic has slowed to the lowest level in centuries. The slowdown of the Gulf Stream devastates fisheries and will lead to a rise in sea levels.

Desertification on 2/3 of all the land on earth
TED presentation Allan Savory.
https://youtu.be/vpTHi7O66pI

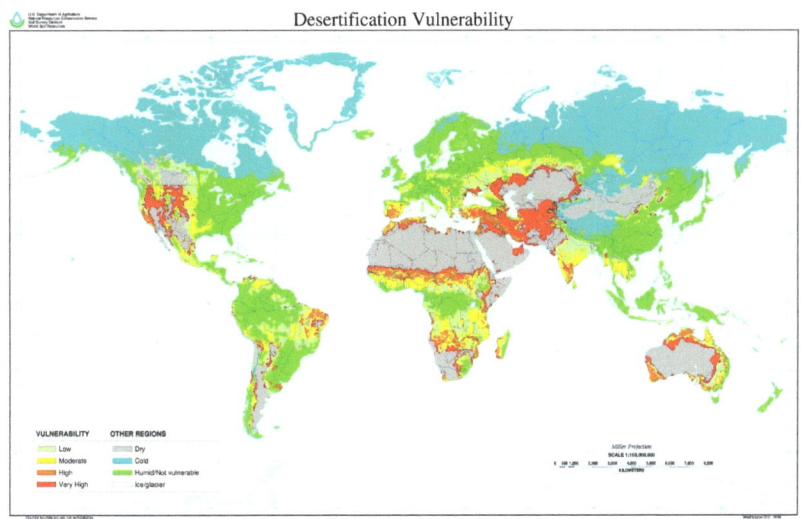

- When humans mastered fire, language and developed weapons like spears and axes, they were formidable predators. This was especially the case in the grasslands where their prey ran in herds. The grasslands with their deep, water and carbonaceous soils had developed for millions of years thanks to the balance between grazing animals, and the predators that fed with them.

- Modern farming methods contribute significantly to desertification and climate change due to water and air pollution from agriculture and intensive breeding of pigs, poultry and livestock. By breaking down agricultural land, we are reducing its enormous ability to retain and contain carbon.

- Chemical fertilizers to increase production have killed microorganisms in the soil, reduced fertility of the soil and the ability to retain water and led to additional flooding. Pesticides used for the treatment of internal parasites in animals have led to the destruction of dung beetles, which are vital for soil renewal.

- Fires break the ground cover in a way that it easily carries away by rain and wind. Huge man-made deserts have arisen. According NASA pictures from space about two thirds of the land is deserted.

- Banks finance the farmers to rent out their pastures for solar panels and windmills and to set up even more megafarms with the aid of electrical energy.

An ever-growing meat production causes drought and hunger in large parts of the world. Fast food and an increase in meat consumption in the West are also being imitated in other parts of the world. Modern agriculture makes an important contribution to desertification and climate change due to water and air pollution from agriculture and intensive breeding of pigs, poultry and livestock. By demolishing agricultural land, we reduce the enormous ability of land to hold carbon.

Wildlife loss

- In the last 50 years homo sapiens has wiped out 60% of mammals, birds, fish and reptiles in the wild
- Humankind has destroyed 83% of all mammals and half of plants since the dawn of civilization.
- Wildlife hunting in tropical forests reduces bird and mammal populations.

Humans and our ancestors have likely consumed bushmeat, wild animals killed for food. During the 20th century, however, commercial hunting using firearms and wire snares to supply logging and oil exploration concessions along new roadway networks has dramatically increased the catch in Central African forests. Annually, it is estimated that 579 million wild animals are caught and consumed in the Congo basin, equaling 4.5 million tons of bushmeat, with the addition of a possible 5 million tons of wild mammalian meat from the Amazon basin. Tropical lowland forest habitat contains the world's greatest terrestrial biodiversity and may therefore harbor a reservoir of zoonotic pathogens. The wildlife trade in general generates in excess one billion direct and indirect contacts between humans and domesticated animals annually. The broad range of tissue and fluid exposures associated with the bush meat industry's hunting and butchering may take these wildlife interactions especially risky. In Africa, as many as 30 different species of primates are also hunted and processed by the bushmeat industry.

- The increase in meat products and dairy production in the West could only be achieved with artificial insemination of livestock and the animals unilaterally fattening with soy flour, corn and fish meal.

- One billion people suffer from hunger, while 70 billion animals are fattened and eaten every year.
- During the ice ages the Cro-Magnon man was forced to eat more meat because there were fewer grains, fruit, nuts and seeds. Will modern man start eating more fruit and vegetables now that the earth is warming up?
- We can no longer ignore the impact of current unsustainable production models. If we start eating less meat, the farmers can gradually switch from intensive livestock farming to agriculture

Benítez-López A, Alkemade R, Schipper AM et al. The impact of hunting on tropical mammal and bird populations. Science 2017 356(6334):180-183

Overpopulation

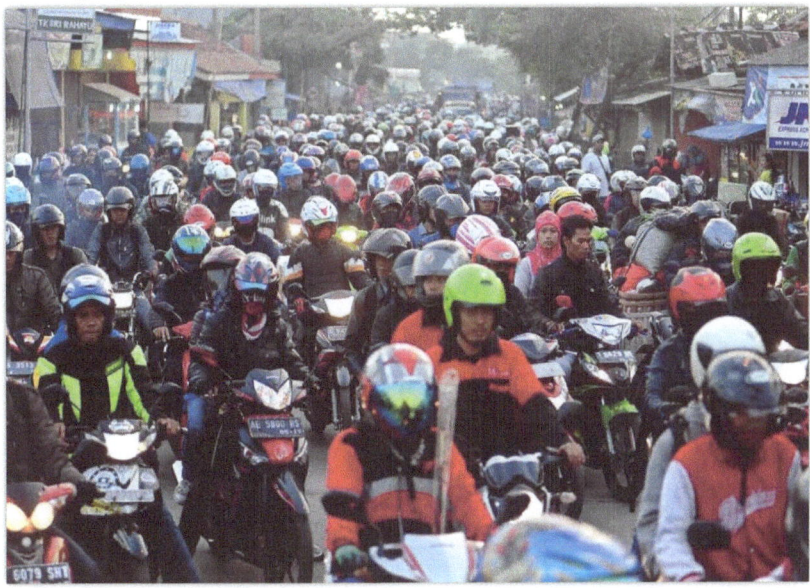

- For example, Indonesia. Half of the population is younger than 15 years.
- Young people take care of the elderly. Many children can take care of their retirement in the absence of a pension.
- When prosperity increased in Europe, the dependence on the elderly decreased and the population increase declined.
- Less prosperous countries can earn income by producing their own food with the new cultivation techniques.

In Singapore, the two-children policy began in the 1970s. Due to the enormous influx of immigrants, the population grew, but the indigenous population growth decreased. The one-child policy of China led to a population reduction of three hundred million people.

Countries with still extreme population growth are Brazil (fifty million inhabitants in 1950, more than two hundred ten million in 2018) and Indonesia (Java in 1960 sixty million inhabitants, one hundred and sixty million in 2018). Africa, now good for one fifth of the world's population, will be the only continent whose population will continue to grow after 2050. The UN expects that by 2100 40 percent of the world will be Africans.

- **If free contraception could be provided to women in Africa, who want to continue learning and work hard for more prosperity for their families, the increase in the population may also decrease here.**

The European population is shrinking. In Singapore, the two-child policy began in the 1970s. The population grew because of the enormous influx of immigrants, but the native population growth declined. China's one-child policy led to a population restriction of three hundred million people. Birth control is most common in China, with 83% of the population using one of the available contraceptives. Slightly less in Europe: 77% - and in North and South America 75%. In Africa, the percentage is shockingly low in some countries. Contraception is expected to increase by 2030 from 17 to 27 percent in West Africa, from 23 to 34 percent in Central Africa, from 40 to 55 percent in East Africa, and from 39 to 45 percent in Melanesia, Micronesia and Polynesia (Trends in contraceptive use worldwide, 2015 United Nations).

Hydrogen as energy source offers the solution

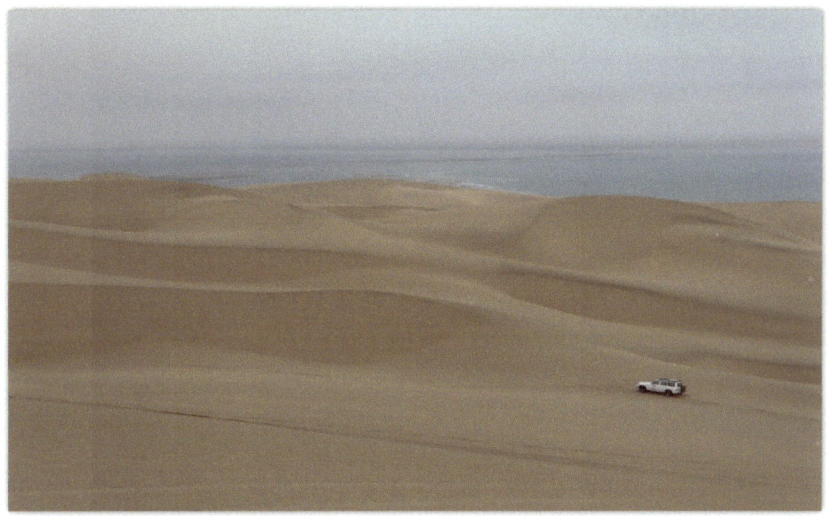

We will be saying goodbye not only to fossil fuels, but also to biofuels. The demand for palm oil has risen so much what is largely due to western policy to stimulate the use of biofuels. The cosmetics and food industries are also major customers. Fires has become increasingly fierce in recent years in the Brazilian Amazon forest and in the Indonesian tropical rainforests of Borneo and Papua New Guinea. The 'slash and burn' method (felling and burning) is used to cultivate natural land for palm plantations. Hydrogen as prime energy source is the solution.

- The Namib desert at Lüderitz, a port on the Atlantic Ocean on the south-west coast of Namibia, is one of the sunniest places in the world. This desert is 200 km wide and extends 2000 km from Angola in the North to the Orange River in the South along the Atlantic Ocean. In this 81,000 km2 a suitable

area for energy production can be found. A combination of solar panels and hydrogen gas production with transport to the sea can offer economic benefits to poor Namibia.
https://youtu.be/a04JKguARZA

- Let Groningen earn from the transition to hydrogen gas. The Netherlands already has an extensive gas network from Groningen to the rest of the Netherlands. This natural gas network can be used for hydrogen gas transport without too much adaptation so that most domestic and industrial connections can use hydrogen gas for heating, cooking and industrial use.

- Veendam has the first larger hydrogen plant in the Netherlands that uses solar power. It is an important step in Groningen's mission to develop into the hydrogen province of the Netherlands. Renewable energy from the electricity grid and 5,000 solar panels on the site provide green electricity to the plant, which can convert one megawatt of sustainable electricity into hydrogen. A hydrogen industry in Groningen can supply the large amounts of energy that will be lost when the oil and gas era is closed. Hydrogen can be stored in empty salt caverns on the EnergyStock site. If all the salt caverns on the site are filled with hydrogen, that will be enough to heat all the houses in the Netherlands for several weeks.

- Researchers from the University of Waterloo in Canada have developed a new fuel cell that lasts at least ten times longer than current technology. These fuel cells can produce electricity from the chemical reaction, when hydrogen and oxygen are combined to make water, and will therefore be much

cheaper. If these fuel cells are mass-produced, they will be able to power hydrogen-gas hybrid vehicles.
http://www.uwaterloo.ca

- Canadian engineers have found a way to produce hydrogen relatively easily and cheaply. By injecting oxygen into the tar sands, the temperature in the soil appears to rise. As a result, hydrogen gas is released from the oil, which can be separated from other gases by special membrane filters. The procedure works in tar sands, but also exhausted and discarded oil fields: wherever there is still oil in the ground that can be heated, leading to the formation of hydrogen gas. Even with oil fields that are still in use, this technique can be used. A polluting fossil resource can thus be given a new lease of life and produce the energy carrier of the future. Hydrogen production is a cost-effective alternative to energy production from oil fields and tar sands. By placing hydrogen filter membranes in the production sources, only the hydrogen is extracted and undesirable by-products such as carbon dioxide diode and methane remain in the soil.
- The existing infrastructure and distribution channels around the oil fields would suffice, keeping production costs low. At the moment it costs about 2 dollars to produce a kilo of H2, but with the new method that would only be 10 to 50 cents. The necessary oxygen can be produced on site. This requires no more than 5 percent of the energy produced.
- The oil sands deposits in Western Canada not only represent a vast store of hydrocarbons (oil) that can be converted into fuel and petrochemicals but also a vast hydrogen store – a super clean valuable energy vector and chemical feedstock. Oil

sands reservoirs that have low energy and emissions intensities, hydrogen production are a viable alternative for energy production from heavy oil and oil sands reservoirs by using in situ gasification technology. Gasification reactions, together with the water-gas shift reaction, enable the generation of hydrogen from both bitumen and water within the oil sands reservoir. With hydrogen separation membranes in the production wells, other products from the reactions remain in the reservoir.

- Researchers at the Lawrence Berkeley National Laboratory (LBL) in California have developed a new type of solar cell. It is a so-called hybrid photovoltaic cell that can produce both electricity and hydrogen. Solar panels with these convert electricity that has not been taken from them into hydrogen during the day, and store it. After all, a fuel cell can be used to convert hydrogen into electricity in the hours when there is no sunlight or when there is a very high demand, as a back-up. The HPEV solar panels (Hybrid Photo Electrochemical and Voltaic) increase efficiency in the generation and use of green electricity and can therefore contribute to achieving a lower price for green hydrogen. This is one of the biggest challenges at the moment, because the production of hydrogen from natural gas is even much cheaper. The HPEV- panels also have a third electrode for converting CO_2. The HPEV-panels have a third electrode, which uses the maximum possible number of electrons to generate hydrogen. The other two electrodes are used to generate electricity, just like conventional solar panels. The researchers are investigating whether this technology could also be used, for example, to remove CO_2 from the air and convert it into usable chemical applications. In any case, it seems that a new type of solar panel is in the making.

- In Stad aan het Haringvliet, The Netherlands, houses are being built with a system for storing solar energy in green hydrogen. This creates the entire chain of sustainable and renewable energy production, storage and use in the living environment. The solar energy from the summer period is stored for use in the winter months (seasonal storage). The gas network of the village can be switched to hydrogen with little cost and inconvenience for residents. The fifteen-kilometer gas network at Stad aan 't Haringvliet is flushed with nitrogen to remove natural gas. `The four gas district stations will be adjusted and the gas pipes in the homes will be checked. The natural gas central heating boilers are replaced by a hydrogen boiler. (www.solencopower.com)

- The houses are completely self-sufficient in terms of energy requirements. Unique and the future of new construction

Chemical preparation of hydrogen from sodium borohydride

Sodium boron hydride (NaBH 4) is a chemical compound from which hydrogen can be extracted. In combination with fuel cells, electricity can be produced safely and with only water as a residual product. The material is a white powder and a well-known ingredient of washing powders. A Dutch inventor brought sodium boron hydride into contact with very pure water and a catalyst. The result: more than 95% of the theoretically feasible amount of hydrogen is actually extracted. A great success that has since been patented and is being further developed, in collaboration with Technical University Delft. You do need water without ions. It is transported to the filling station in granular form. A machine there makes ultrapure water from tapwater. The ultrapure water is then mixed with the sodium boron hydride, creating a pumpable slurry. The 'slurry' - called H2Fuel - is then filled up, just like you fill up with petrol. However, while you're doing that, you're also filling up with highly diluted hydrochloric acid. This is stored in a separate tank from the H2Fuel. If you want to drive, that hydrochloric acid is mixed with the H2Fuel and hydrogen is released within milliseconds. Not only from the sodium boron hydride, but also from the ultrapure water. The hydrogen then goes to the fuel cell, generating electricity. The reaction also results in a number of residual products, including water from the fuel cell. Some of it is filtered back into ultrapure water and used immediately, because you need more of this water than you can fill up with.

An truck, with only 350 litres of sodium boron hydride can go up and down to Barcelona without refuelling. H2Fuel could also be the solution for storing excess renewable energy (generated by solar panels on sunny days, for example) for days with energy shortages (when it is very cloudy or windless, for example). H2Fuel can then help. But if you're going to refuel later, you'll have to leave the residual products behind. This means that truckers have to drive back and forth: they have to bring sodium boron hydride and dispose of residual products. From a logistical point of view, this is much more complicated and therefore more expensive. In addition, H2Fuel requires considerable modification of the existing (hydrogen) car. After all, you have to have three tanks: one for the sodium boron hydride, one for the diluted hydrochloric acid and one for the spent fuel. The company creates these three tanks by placing partitions in a tank and expects the automotive industry to implement this tank in the near future, but that is still questionable.

- The H2Fuel process, with a very high yield, has already been validated by TNO (www.h2-fuel.nl). Hydrogen gas is not extracted from the ground and can be produced anywhere in the world (www.h2fuel.com).
- H2Fuel, a sodium-borohydride compound, is the carrier of hydrogen. The chemical name is $NaBH_4$ (powder) and can be stored indefinitely under normal atmospheric conditions. To release the hydrogen, Ultra Pure Water (UPW = fully pure H_2O) and a little dilute hydrochloric acid are added in a certain ratio and the hydrogen molecules of both the $NaBH_4$ and H_2O are released. A total of 8H. This high yield of hydrogen molecules is only possible with the use of UPW (patented). With this hydrogen, electricity and / or heat can be produced via a fuel cell.
- $NaBH_4 + 2\ H_2O = 4\ H_2 + NaBO_2$ + heat. The residual product $NaBO_2$ can be converted into $NaBH_4$ in a new chemical process. The energy required for this can be supplied by solar and / or wind energy. The average power of a Dutch windmill is around 1,000 kWh.
- Refueling sodium borohydride at the farmer has advantages over intake at a gas station. Upgrading the residual liquid requires electricity and the combination of electricity and highly flammable fuels at a Shell gas station is undesirable.
- H2Fuel is completely free from any harmful emissions during production, storage, transport and consumption. The environmental tax can then expire in the long term.
- On sea-going vessels osmosis allows UPW to extract fully pure water from seawater and space is available for this type of power plant.

- A Hyundai NEXO is equipped with a 156-liter compression tank (700 bar) with hydrogen gas and has a range of 666 km. The high vehicle weight (1814 kg) comes at the expense of acceleration. With a 60-liter normal tank with sodium borohydride powder slurry, a hydrogen car can be much lighter and have a range of 700 km (2.5 times larger with the same amount of hydrogen).
- The drive system of the Hyundai Nexo delivers a power of 135 kW (184 hp) and with a full tank of hydrogen you can cover approximately 580 kilometres. Taking H2 fuel from the farmer and revaluing the residual liquid will be possible. Great figures for daily use.
- A grant project to speed up the chemical preparation of hydrogen would be great. A greenhouse complex in the Westland wants to be able to produce energy-neutral fruit and vegetables all year round with the help of a hydrogen power plant. Some vans are also converted into hydrogen cars and can refuel at the greenhouse complex and have the residual liquid here upgraded.
- Vertical agriculture and horticulture require a lot of heat, light and space to produce strawberries, lettuce, cauliflower, peppers, grapes and also tropical fruit such as pineapples all year round. Here too, such a power plant with fuel cells can be used. Farmers can give their warehouses a new destination. With local production with a greater supply and diversity, the current supply of fruit and vegetables over the equator will be able to decrease.

Farming transition offers the solution

Vertical farming, multilayer cultivation, also called city farming

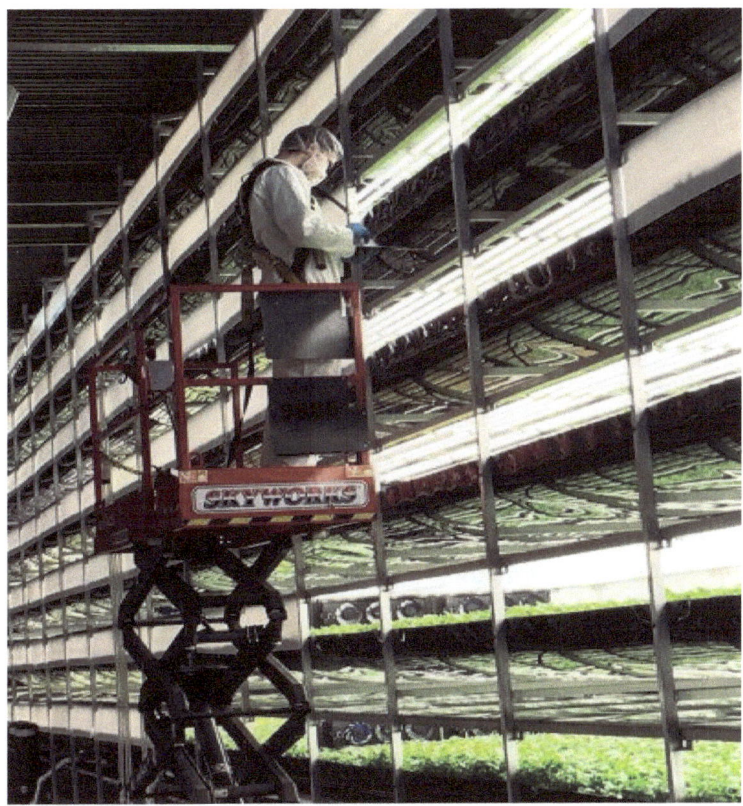

The usual agriculture and horticulture run on artificial fertilizers, pesticides and new plant varieties

- Unsprayed fruit and vegetables, pesticides are no longer needed

- In such a closed system, pests and diseases are no longer a chance

- Growing in two weeks which takes 30 days in the open ground with 95 percent less water consumption, fewer fertilizers, and completely without pesticides.
- Techniques can also be applied outside Europe and the USA.

Sunlight cannot be controlled. And the high-pressure sodium lamps with which Dutch growers provide extra light for their greenhouses can only be used to a limited extent. They give orange / yellow light and are too warm to place near plants. With the cooler LED lamps, which can contain all kinds of colors, engineers can develop a light recipe. They can choose the right combinations of wavelengths and light intensities, place the LED lamps near the plants, and opt for wider or narrower light beams. By altering the color of lights change the smell, taste and even the vitamin content of tomatoes. For more efficient growth, switch on the red light; to develop shorter plants with higher levels of antioxidants, use more blue light.

The reason for the higher yield, compared to greenhouses and outdoor cultivation, is that under LED lighting the entire plant, the whole year and long days can get enough light. In the uncontrolled sunlight, moreover, part is lost because one sheet gets too much and the other gets too little. Light is also lost due to reflection and the falling of photons on the ground. In order to make the collection of light more efficient, companies can drop light beams onto the leaves at certain angles. Or place LED lamps between plants. Strawberries are sweeter and tastier when the leaves and fruit are extra lighted. Dozens of vertical farms, also called 'vegetable factories' or 'indoor farms', supply spinach, bok choy, dill or cabbage every day. In climate-controlled rooms grow in four layers among others grow lettuce, strawberries, coriander and watercress. In an average Dutch greenhouse, the lettuce yield is 60 kilos per square meter of floor per year. 100 kilograms per square meter shelf will be taken in the vertical shelves. In Miyagi, Japan, a Japanese plant physiologist ordered 17,500 LED lamps that had to be installed in a former Sony factory. This factory supplies 10,000 unsprayed lettuce heads per day. In Singapore, Panasonic opened a fully automated indoor farm for 81 tons of vegetables every year. Aero Farms in Newark, USA, opened the largest so far, a nine-meter-high warehouse that will supply 250 different unsprayed vegetables and herbs.

Greenhouses are an area where machines are still surprisingly absent: picking crops such as tomatoes, peppers and strawberries has not yet been spent on robot hands on a large scale. Throughout the year, armies of pickers move into the greenhouses, which usually have relatively low wages and long and arduous working days. The picking robot is already used in Japan. In the absence of cheap labour, farmers there are in some cases satisfied with robots that harvest far less than human pickers. Even if the robot only harvests sixty or seventy percent of all strawberries, the grower earns more than if he hires relatively expensive pickers.

Agriculture on saline soils

- On Texel they succeeded in growing potatoes and vegetables on saline ground.

- Worldwide, 1.5 billion hectares of agricultural land are threatened by salinization. In areas where salinization poses the greatest threat, this offers a chance to feed families independently.
- Can the salty potato save people from the famine? Since 2010, Zilt Proefbedrijf Texel has been researching which crops grow on salty soil. Many species do well.
- The fermentation of seaweed releases 2/3 methane gas and 1/3 hydrogen gas which must only be collected and used better than the alternatives for natural gas that are currently available.

Salty potatoes

The salty potato is creamy and purely organic. Developed on the salty soil of Texel and fertilized with seaweed. As a result, these potatoes are rich in minerals and natural vitamins. This potato can be cooked in the shell. You can also cook them well in oven or frying pan. The taste is recognizable, yet surprisingly different. The most flavorful potato from the Wageningen University taste test! Adding salt is not necessary.

Salty vegetables that are grown on Texel:

- Samphire
- Lamb's lettuce
- Ice-herb
- Sea cabbage stalks and sprouts
- Sea fennel
- Beach beet
- Oyster leaf
- Salty RAF Tomato
- Truffle weed

Let Plant Based Food be the medicine for health

Nutrition as prevention and to support the treatment of cancer. We eat everything that tastes good. If it is cheap and tasty, it also accelerates chronic disease and tumor formation. This is how our food system works. The raw materials for factory preparation are limited. Soy, corn, eggs, refined sugars, animal proteins and trans fats. These are the main ingredients that the largest food companies use to make the food that is all around us. It is not that these big companies do not care. In fact, it is difficult for them to do something else. In parts of the world with less chemical agriculture, less factory food processing, mortality from cancer is lower. Fruits and vegetables contain more bio-active substances.

- Fruits and vegetables make bio-active substances that delay the growth and propagation of intruders.

Plant-based nutrition works life-extending
Voluntary restriction of the diet will probably never gain much popularity as a life-prolonging strategy. Vegetable diets have a low methionine content. Vegetable proteins - especially those from vegetables or nuts - contain less methionine than animal proteins. Several animal studies with methionine restricted diet have shown inhibition of cancer cell growth and prolonged healthy life span in experimental animals. American researchers have looked at 30 years of nutrition data among 130,000 people. They found a reduced risk of premature death in those who ate more vegetable protein and a higher risk in those who ate more animal protein. Each increase of 3% more vegetable proteins in the diet reduced the risk of death, by whatever cause, during the period under review by 10%. A link was also shown with a 12% lower

risk of death from cardiovascular disease. But a 10% higher share of animal proteins in the diet led to a 2% higher risk of death and 8% higher chance of dying of a heart problem (Song M).

Plant-based food is not boring and one-sided. Exotic fruits, herbs, soya and vegetables can very well replace all meat and meat products in our supermarkets. On the land, 250,000 different varieties of plants can be grown and in the oceans there are another 20,000 different species, including seaweed, rich in omega-3 oils. The countries of the southern hemisphere could also make a larger contribution to this. The recipe is still in its infancy.

Animal proteins and vegetable proteins from the oceans are healthier than animal proteins from intensive livestock farming. The oceans offer a good choice of anchovies, mussels, oysters, squid, herring, mackerel, cod, sprat, sole, crabs, lobsters, shrimps and even wild tuna and salmon.

The human body defends against invading bacteria, spores and yeast cells, with the help of antibodies, white blood cells, macrophages and T-cells. The body is unable to produce antioxidants such as beta-carotene, vitamin C and is unable to make vegetable bio-active substances. Unnatural nutrition is the cause of deficits and chronic diseases. Fast food, many meat products and little fruit and vegetables weaken the natural defenses. The question remains how a revolution in public opinion can be achieved in order to massively switch exclusively to natural food with supplementing necessary supplements for existing shortages.

Vitamin C

Not so long ago during the great voyages of discovery, it has already been discovered that vitamin C deficiencies arise due to lack of fresh fruit and vegetables. This gave the sailors scurvy with internal bleeding, which usually resulted in death. Vitamin C is necessary for the construction of connective tissue proteins. Deficient production of these connective tissue proteins weakens the blood vessels with bleeding as a result. Due to the frequent use of pesticides in agriculture, the content of bioactive antibodies in fruit and vegetables has been reduced, as a result of which our defense against cell infections is even more affected.

Vitamin D

Sufficient vitamin D increases bone density, which means less chance of bone fractures. Vitamin D is not really a vitamin, but the precursor of the powerful steroid hormone calcitrol, which has widespread actions throughout the body. Several studies have shown that vitamin D deficiency increases the risk of developing cancer and that avoiding a deficiency and adding vitamin D supplements can be an economical and safe way to reduce the incidence of cancer and the prognosis and result of cancer treatment. Vitamin D is a fat-soluble vitamin and is sold as pearl capsules. Vitamin supra D3 forte capsules (Bayer) contain 20 mcg equivalent to 800 IU. If a deficiency has been established, at least 2 pearls per day should be taken.

Coconut oil

Coconut oil is a vegetable fat that is well processed by the body. The grease already melts at a temperature of 24 degrees Celsius and is resistant to high temperatures. Coconut fat is very suitable for baking and roasting. One or two coffee spoons (5-10 ml) is sufficient. When firing for frying and roasting, less combustion products form than when heating the other vegetable oils, sunflower oil and olive oil. It promotes the absorption of the fat-soluble vitamins A-D-E and K. Vegetable fat contains nutrients for nerve and brain cells. Overweight and diabetes mellitus are common in later life. For these risk groups it has been demonstrated that the use of 40 ml coconut fat per day has a beneficial effect. When the body produces too little insulin, the energy supply (glucose) to the brain is jeopardized. Coconut fat promotes an alternative energy supply to the brain cells after admission. Coconut oil has a beneficial effect on the energy intake of brain cells and memory loss in Alzheimer's disease (De la Rubia Orti 2017).

Curcuma

Curcuma, a natural polyphenol compound, isolated from the rhizome of a herbaceous perennial plant, has anticancer activity. We need to consume a sufficient amount of bio-active substances with fruit and vegetables to keep out invaders. Bioactive antibodies inhibit the overactivity of the enzyme CYP1B1 in cancer cells. Infected or damaged cells are now seen as abnormal and are removed from the body by growth inhibition and the death of the infected cell.

Benefits of Mediterranean food

The diet in Spain, Italy and Greece is one of the healthiest eating habits in the world. There are apparently fewer diseases here, and mortality from some chronic diseases is also less. This dietary pattern is rich in fruit and vegetables, fish and less saturated fat containing dairy products. This eating habit reduces the risk of cardiovascular disease, reduces the risk of diabetes, prolongs the lifespan and counts more healthy elderly people.

Avoid fast food

Old McDonald's farm is very different than the McDonald of today. Fast food is in fashion. Hamburgers and chicken burgers are often on the menu of hard-working people. It is no longer rare for someone to go to bed with a bag of chips. Vegetables, fruit and herbs contain more antibodies, antioxidants and vitamin C. Green vegetables, artichokes, asparagus, cabbage, peppers, avocados, carrots, celery, cucumber, spinach, pumpkin, courgettes and aubergines are all important sources of antibodies. Fruits, especially red fruits such as berries, grapes, apples, strawberries, prunes, figs, raspberries, mandarins, oranges, pears, melon, pineapple, mango and olives contain antibodies. Herbs contain a high content of bio-active substances in parsley, basil, rosemary, thyme, sage, mint and rose hips.

Avoid unhealthy trans fats

Vegetable (unsaturated) fats are liquid at room temperature and can only be processed by the food industry as a solid substance. These fats are converted into partially hardened fat by a chemical process. Products that contain partially hydrogenated fats and trans fatty acids, such as margarine, chips, cookies, coffee milk powder, tarts, crackers and pizzas are bad for blood vessels. Nowadays, croissants are often made with hydrogenated vegetable oils instead of butter. Cheap mass production means that a croissant contains more fat (17 grams), which consists of about one third (5 to 6 grams) of trans fats.

It is difficult and often impossible to escape the temptations of major industrial interests.

- Light products are the answer of the sugar industry. Fats are replaced by sugars by the food industry, which has a counterproductive effect and makes us eat more.
- The electronic cigarette is the answer of the tobacco industry to get rid of cigarette addicts.
- The vegaburger is the answer of the food industry to the consumer, who no longer wants meat, to meet our addiction to meat products and hamburgers.

References cardiovascular disease and type 2 diabetes

Arcari CM, Gaydos CA, Nieto FJ, Krauss M, Nelson KE (2005) Association between Chlamydia pneumoniae Immunoglobulin A and acute myocardial infarction in young men in the United States military: importance of timing of exposure measurements. Clin Infect Dis 40:1123-30

Bodai BI, Nakata TE, Wong WT et al. Lifestyle Medicine: A Brief Review of Its Dramatic Impact on Health and Survival. Perm J 2017;22
https://www.ncbi.nlm.nih.gov/pubmed/29035175

Belland RJ, Ouellette SP, Gieffers J, Byrne GI. (2004) Chlamydia pneumoniae and atherosclerosis. Cell Microbiol. 2004 Feb;6(2):117-27.

Campbell TC, Parpia B, Chen J (1998) Diet, lifestyle, and the etiology of coronary artery disease: the Cornell China study. Am J Cardiol. Nov 26;82(10B):18T-21T.

Campbell TC, Campbell TM (2006) The China Study. e-Book Apple.

Cavuoto P, Fenech MF (2012) A review of methionine dependency and the role of methionine restriction in cancer growth control and life-span extension. Cancer Treat Rev. 2012 Oct;38(6):726-36

Contini C, Seraceni S, Cultrera R et al. (2010) Chlamydophila pneumoniae Infection and Its Role in Neurological Disorders. Interdiscip Perspect Infect Dis. 2010: 273573 Section of Infectious Diseases, Department of Clinical and Experimental Medicine, University of Ferrara, Italy.

De la Rubia Orti JE (2017) How does coconut oil affect cognitive performance in Alzheimer patients? A prospective clinical trial in region Valencia. Nutr. Hosp. 352

Deshazo RD, Bigler S, Skipworth LB. (2013) The autopsy of chicken nuggets reads "chicken little". Am J Med. 2013 Nov;126(11):1018-9.

Esselstyn CB Jr, Ellis SG, Medendorp SV, et al. A strategy to arrest and reverse coronary artery disease: a 5-year longitudinal study of a single physician's practice. J Fam Pract. 1995;41:560-568

Esselstyn CB Jr. Is the present therapy for coronary artery disease the radical mastectomy of twenty-first century? Am J Cardiol 2010;106:902-904

Esselstyn CB Jr, Gendy G, Doyle J, Golubic M, Roizen MF (2014) A way to reverse CAD? J Fam Pract. 2014 Jul;63(7):356-364b

Grayston JT: Chlamydia pneumoniae, atherosclerosis and coronary heart disease (CHD). Clin Infect Dis 2005, 40:1131-1132

Holst PAJ (2015) Plant-Based food is your Best Medicine to avoid chronic diseases and cancer. e-book APPLE 106 pages ISBN 978-90-822105-6-9

Holst PAJ (2016) Vegetarian Food everyday keeps your doctor away E-book APPLE 144pages

Holst PAJ (2016) The Blueprint of Cancer, how to change your lifestyle and eating habits. e-book 234 pages ISBN 97890822105-9-0

Peter Holst MD PhD (2016) PREVENTION IS BETTER THAN CURE is Bad News for meat industry, tobacco industry, fast food industry and pharmaceutical industry. BOL.com E-book 978-90-824963-2-1

Khaw KT, Sharp SJ, Finikarides L, Afzal I, Lentjes M, Luben R, Forouhi NG. Randomised trial of coconut oil, olive oil or butter on blood lipids and other cardiovascular risk factors in healthy men and women. BMJ Open. 2018 Mar 6;8(3):e020167.
https://bmjopen.bmj.com/content/8/3/e020167

Song M, Fung TT, Hu FB, Willett WC, Longo VD, Chan AT, Giovannucci EL (2016) Association of Animal and Plant Protein Intake With All-Cause and Cause- Specific Mortality. JAMA Intern Med. 2016 Aug 1

Wang Y, Yu H, Zhang X et al. Evaluation of daily ginger consumption for the prevention of chronic diseases in adults: A cross-sectional study. Nutrition. 2017 Apr;36:79-84.

Simply make your own meals

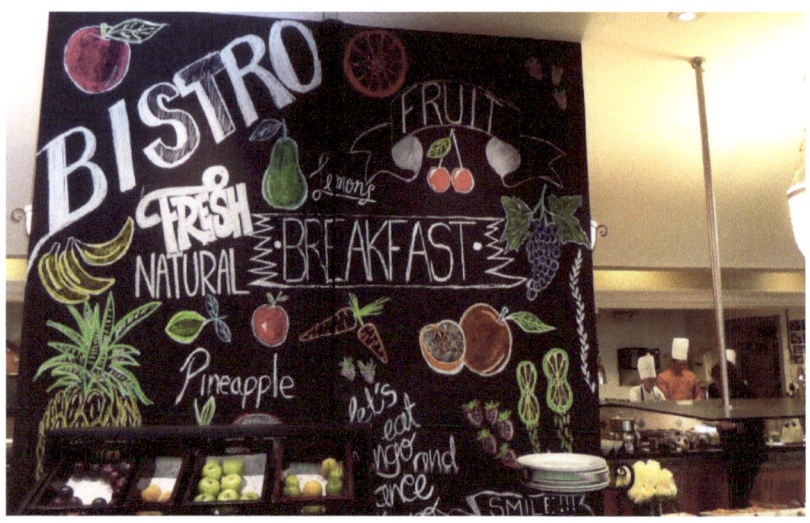

Stick to this simple advice to get rid of excess body fat and prevent diseases. Avoid white bread, white pasta, white rice, potatoes, French fries, breakfast cake, egg cakes, chips, honey, baguette and beer to lose weight faster. Nutrition must contain many vegetables, but also sufficient vegetable proteins and fats (fish, olive oil, avocado, etc.).

Start with a plant-based diet, and the need for animal proteins and fats will gradually decline

In addition to diet, physical activity and extra antioxidant intake may counteract DNA methylation changes contributing to aging.

Fruit Breakfast

Start with two glasses of water

Oatmeal flakes with broken flax seed in soy yoghurt or soya light, almond milk or coconut milk.

With fresh fruit. like strawberries, raspberries, apples, pear, mandarin, orange, melon etc. Cut the fruit into pieces to preserve the dietary fiber.

Soup with the lunch

Make soup from vegetable broth. Think of tomato, vegetable, onion, pumpkin, mushroom, broccoli soup. A delicious soup can be made of all vegetables.

Salad with nuts, mushrooms, arugula, tomato, onion, garlic, green beans, kidney beans, chickpeas etc. Mix your salad with plenty olive oil.

Sandwich with salad of tuna, salmon, shrimp etc. or an omelet or hard-boiled egg. Omega-3 rich fish such as salmon, herring, mackerel and shellfish like mussels are much healthier than red meat.

- *No sausages, hard-boiled eggs only, no meat (products) from the super, no insufficiently cooked BBQ meat, less dairy products, no raw milk cheese.*

Hot meal

Make especially use of herbs and spices. Replace the meat you were used to for example with chickpeas, brown or white beans. Use olives and nuts. Make a delicious chili sin carne or curry dish with cauliflower, broccoli and chickpeas.

Bake and roast with coconut fat or olive oil

Coconut fat is very suitable for baking and roasting. Melt a coffee spoon (5 ml) in the pan is sufficient. When heating and roasting, less combustion products form than when heating the other vegetable oils, sunflower and olive oil.

No dessert

Avoid in case of excess weight sugars and quickly digestible carbohydrates. More healthy fats give a feeling of satiety and forces the liver to burn absorbed fats and belly fats when energy is required by the body. By sweetening, the liver chooses the path of least resistance (glycolysis) and provides the requested energy, glucose, and stores excess to body fat.

Drink black coffee, green tea or ginger tea after the meal. Ginger tea can be made by cutting slices from ginger root and letting it boil in boiling water.

- *Alcohol and wine in moderation. The degradation product acetaldehyde is harmful to our DNA. Too many wine acids damage the esophagus and stomach.*

Your Target Weight

The abdominal circumference around the navel in relation to body height is a good measure of (over) weight. Belt length 93 cm divided by body length 186 cm = 0.5 should preferably be less than 50%

Men	Women	
< 35%	< 35%	Underweight
35% - 45%	35% - 42%	Extremely Slim
43% - 46%	42% - 46%	Healthy
46%– 53%	46% - 49%	Normal Weight
53% - 58%	49% - 54%	Overweight
58% - 63%	54% - 58%	Obese
> 63%	> 58%	Highly Obese

Burning Belly Fat

Fat burning only starts after twenty minutes of exercise. Until this time of 20 minutes, especially carbohydrate reserves (the glycogen in the liver and muscles) are burned and you will not lose weight. This means that you start the fat burning process during the last part of the training. That is why it is better to exercise for one hour three times a week (3 x 40 minutes fat burning) than six times a week for half an hour (6 x 10 minutes fat burning). It does not matter what the training consists of. This can be brisk walking, slow jogging or a session on a treadmill or rowing machine.

References

The National Center for Biotechnology Information (NCBI) was established in 1988 as a department of the National Institutes of Health. NIH was selected for their experience in creating and maintaining biomedical databases. The collection of research reports from NIH represent the largest biomedical research facility in the world.
All the studies mentioned in this book can be consulted on the internet page of the NCBI by entering the matching database number.
For example:Is breast cancer a zoonosis?
Szabo S, Haislip AM, Garry RF (2005) Of mice, cats, and men: is human breast cancer a zoonosis? Microsc Res Tech. 68(3-4):197-208. Review

https://www.ncbi.nlm.nih.gov/pubmed/16276516

Malignant lymphomas and Chlamydia pneumoniae infections
Chronic infections can predict malignant growth. A connection has been shown of chronic Chlamydia pneumoniae infection with lung cancer. In the study of Anttila TI an association was found between chronic C. pneumoniae infections and malignant lymphomas (Anttila TI). The link was most present with Non-Hodgkin lymphoma (OR = 7.3, 95% CI 2.2 to 25).25)

Healing of malignant lymphoma with doxycycline
Chlamydia psittaci (Cp), the bacterium of psittacose has often been shown in malignant lymphomas. The bacterium has been shown in the tumor tissue, taken out and cell cultures are made. By treatment with doxycycline malignant lymphomas are cured (Ferreri AJ).

Ferreri AJ, Dolcetti R, Magnino S ey al. (2007) A woman and her canary: a tale of chlamydiae and lymphomas. J Natl Cancer Inst. 2007 Sep 19;99(18):1418-9
https://www.ncbi.nlm.nih.gov/pubmed/17848672

Treatment with doxycycline (twice daily 100 mg) for six months disappeared the malignant lymphomas in 64% of patients. Tetracycline and macrolide (erythromycin) antibiotics have a remarkable therapeutic effect on Cp infection. Cp infection is thus controllable. Chlamydiae have no cell wall and, like viruses, are completely dependent on their host cells. Once in the host cell, Chlamydiae is not sensitive to penicillin. Tetracycline enters cells in the contaminated body cells by diffusion along membrane pores. Once in the cell, tetracyclines and doxycycline inhibit internal cell metabolism, DNA and protein synthesis, whereby Chlamydia cell parasites cannot create new proteins for growth and proliferation.

Anttila TI, Lehtinen T, Leinonen M, Bloigu A, Koskela P, Lehtinen M, Saikku P (1998) Serological evidence of an association between chlamydial infections and malignant lymphomas. Br J Haematol. Oct;103(1):150-6.

https://www.ncbi.nlm.nih.gov/pubmed/9792302

Ferreri AJ 2005, Ponzoni M, Guidoboni M et al. Regression of ocular adnexal lymphoma after Chlamydia psittaci-eradicating antibiotic therapy. J Clin Oncol 2005, 23:5067–5073.

Ferreri AJ, Ponzoni M, Guidoboni M et al. (2006) Bacteria-eradicating therapy with doxycycline in ocular adnexal MALT lymphoma: a multicenter prospective trial. J Natl Cancer Inst 98:1375– 1382.

https://www.ncbi.nlm.nih.gov/pubmed/15968003

Ferreri AJ, Govi S, Pasini E et al. (2012) Chlamydophila Psittaci Eradication with Doxycycline as first-line targeted therapy for Ocular Adnexae Lymphoma: Final Results of an International Phase II Trial. J Clin Oncol 3

https://www.ncbi.nlm.nih.gov/pubmed/22802315

More books from this author

Holst PAJ (1987), Pet birds and hazards to health. Eburon ISBN 90-70879-76-X Delft

Holst PAJ (1991), Birdkeeping as a Source of Lung Cancer and Other Human Diseases. A Need for Higher Hygienic Standards. Springer-Verlag ISBN 3-540- 53555-1, Berlin/Heidelberg Springer-Verlag ISBN 3-387-53555-1, New York

Holst PAJ (2013) Caged birds and laying hens can cause cancer in man. E-book APPLE ISBN 978-90-818776-7-1
paperback ISBN 978-94-021119-0-02

Peter Holst MD PhD (2014) The Last Chimpanzee, somewhere in the 21st century, the last chimpanzee will die. E-book APPLE
paperback ISBN 978-94-02124-8-4

Holst PAJ (2015) Plant-Based food is your Best Medicine to avoid chronic diseases and cancer. E-book APPLE 106 pages ISBN 9789082210569

Holst PAJ (2016) Vegetarian Food everyday keeps your doctor away E-book APPLE 144 pages

Peter Holst MD PhD (2016) **Common Cancers are Zoonoses**
E-book APPLE 197 pages ISBN 978-90-824963-3-8

Peter A.J. Holst MD PhD (2016) Increase in Cancer is a Recent Event.
E-book Apple ISBN 978-90-824963-0-7

Peter Holst MD PhD (2016) PREVENTION IS BETTER THAN CURE is Bad News for meat industry, tobacco industry, fast food industry and pharmaceutical industry.
E-book 978-90-824963-2-1

Holst PAJ (2016) The **Blueprint of Cancer**, how to change your lifestyle and eating habits. e-book 234 pages ISBN 978-90-822105-9-0

Peter A.J. Holst MD PhD (2018) Bye Bye Meat Industry
E-book APPLE 110 pages ISBN 978-90-827267-3-2

Peter A.J. Holst MD PhD (2019) Stop the Meatballs and prepare your own meals.
Paperback 131 pages ISBN 978-1797658926

Peter A.J. Holst MD PhD (2019) Our Inheritance from the Great Apes.
Paperback. 146 pages ISBN 978-1081342159

www.ingramcontent.com/pod-product-compliance
Lightning Source LLC
Chambersburg PA
CBHW040219220526
45473CB00001B/45